MW01279868

PACING

YOURSELF

Steps To Help Save Your Energy

by

Diane Christy, M.S.

and

Carol A. Sarafconn, OTR/L

accent press

Accent Special Publications
Cheever Publishing, Inc.
Post Office Box 700
Bloomington, IL 61702

Cheever Publishing, Inc. serves disabled persons by
collecting and disseminating specialized information.
Services are available through ACCENT on Living,
a quarterly magazine; Accent On Information, a
computerized retrieval system; and Accent Special
Publications.

First Edition
First Printing, October 1990

Library of Congress Catalog Card Number: 90-84915

ISBN 0-915708-31-0

Printed in the United States of America

There is an increasing number and variety of products becoming available to help people with physical limitations perform everyday tasks. ACCENT On Information (AOI) is a computerized information retrieval system that was set up to make it easy to get information about these special products. AOI can provide you with a variety of information on products and where to get them. Write to AOI, P.O. Box 700, Bloomington, IL 61702 to get a search request form or to request information about a specific product.

CONTENTS

Start The Day The Night Before • Keep Ahead Of
Housekeeping • Choose A Wardrobe To Fit Your
Energy Budget

Delegation Is A Key To Conserving Energy • Planning
Can Save Energy • Sit To Work Whenever Possible •
Organizing Space Is A Key To Conserving Energy

Days For Errands • Group Errands Geographically
• Find And Use Delivery Services • The Telephone Is
Man's Best Friend • Use Carrying Aids

Humor Can Go A Long Way • Unclutter And Redirect
Traffic • Designate A Room According To Usage, Not
Convention • Landscape For Low Maintenance • Liv-
ing With Others Can Lead To Greater Independence

Good Posture Saves Energy • Effective Body Mechanics Make Moving Things Easier And Safer • Flexibility

*In loving dedication to my parents, whose
sacrifice, patience, love and laughter
taught that no hurdle was insurmountable.
— D.C.*

*To my grandmothers who adapt gracefully.
— C.A.S.*

INTRODUCTION

by Diane Christy, M.S.

Many people are troubled by a low energy level and the daily frustration, exhaustion and depression that goes along with it. Endurance can be reduced by aging, a heart condition, arthritis, a chronic disease, respiratory ailments, or any number of other conditions. Whatever the origin and whatever the age, life's quality does not have to be anything less than desired. Compromises can be balanced with ultimate joys.

My life-long medical condition leaves me with so little energy, that a walk around the block spells dangerous exhaustion. In spite of this, I parent an energetic nine-year-old boy. I do the cooking, housekeeping, and carpooling, as well as professional writing and lecturing. For years I worked a demanding, full-time job, after completing college and graduate school. All of this is managed by carefully pacing myself.

It takes planning to achieve a balance of necessary and enjoyable activities, while avoiding over exertion. However, when I must adjust for unplanned events or unanticipated fatigue or pain, this balance helps and the planning pays off. Days become tapestries — intricate weavings of rests and planned activities, each with a special method or trick.

The energy-saving methods I use come from years of personal experience, from my family and friends, and from my work as a genetic counselor. Frequently my patients needed energy conservation help, so together we planned and devised methods to meet their needs. Our ideas included organizing the home to cut down on household work, streamlining personal care, building endurance, kitchen short-cuts, "help-visits" to accomplish difficult tasks and even how to foster intimate relationships.

After the years of learning and accumulation of information, it seemed a natural outgrowth for me to compile all of this into a book. I wanted others with reduced or declining energy to have a single resource that was practical, informative and easily related to. The reader will hopefully be able to personally tailor the information and expand and improve upon the ideas presented.

My co-author, Carol Sarafconn, is an experienced teacher who returned to college, after raising her children, to study occupational therapy. Occupational therapists often work with people who have to adjust, some quite suddenly, to lowered energy levels. They teach their clients how to simplify their work and conserve energy.

Our combined personal and professional experiences have taught us that a little energy goes a long way. By planning and pacing yourself, you can accomplish the things that are important to you. You can decrease energy wasted on routine tasks by re-arranging your home and your habits. Learning when to say "no" helps avoid dangerous exhaustion and makes it possible to say "yes" another time. Through improved communication and the use of various techniques, a new physical and emotional intimacy can be brought into your life. And by knowing when to ask for help, you can save your strength for the things only you can do.

We hope this handbook will be a companion in your quest for a personal balance. It is also our hope that teachers, health professionals, families and friends will find *Pacing Yourself* a valuable resource.

The A.M. Shuffle — 1

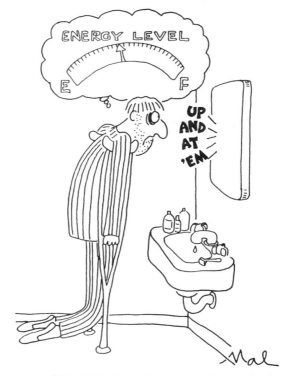

START THE DAY THE NIGHT BEFORE

KEEP AHEAD OF HOUSEKEEPING

CHOOSE A WARDROBE TO FIT YOUR ENERGY BUDGET

PERSONAL CARE
AND STARTING THE DAY

Some mornings when the alarm goes off, I lie in the dark and think about getting up and dressed. I think about everything I need to do during the day and the people who are counting on me. And I feel so overwhelmed; I start to cry.

For someone with low energy levels, starting the day can be daunting. It is easy to feel frustrated when the simple act of getting dressed begins a vicious cycle. But it is for this very reason that good energy conservation principles should be applied to your activities right from the start. By planning ahead and adjusting your personal care routines a little, you will be able to face the challenges of the day with a smile.

START THE DAY THE NIGHT BEFORE

Get enough sleep. Honestly assess how many hours of sleep you need to be at your best. Set a bedtime accordingly and stick to it. Some people find that by getting up earlier, they actually feel less tired. By allowing extra time for their morning routine, they feel less rushed. Tasks can be done at a more leisurely pace with short respites in between. Sometimes rising before the rest of the household gives you a head start, some time to attend to your own needs before things become more hectic.

The typical American lifestyle calls for most personal care chores to be done first thing in the morning. In a sustained whirlwind of activity one showers, shampoos, brushes teeth, uses the toilet, shaves or applies make-up, blow dries hair, and gets dressed. If you have low energy levels, that is too much to expect of yourself all at once. Start the day that way and you'll be exhausted before breakfast.

Which of your chores could be done the night before? Personal care tasks are traditionally done upon rising, but they all don't have to be. Something as simple as laying out your clothes and medical supplies the night before may streamline your morning routine. Keeping yourself clean and well-groomed is important to both your health and a positive self-image; so don't neglect your personal care tasks, but spread them out. Do some the night before, some first thing in the morning, and some later in the day.

Could any of your personal care chores be done less frequently or eliminated altogether? A daily shower and shampoo is a fairly new American habit and one that takes a lot of energy. Consider showering less often and washing up at the sink in between. Men, do you need to shave every day? What about a beard? Women, do you need to shave? Do you need make-up? Each of us will answer these questions differently; but do consider the possibility that longstanding self-care habits may not be the only way to look and feel good. If you have low energy levels, you already know that each day is full of trade-offs. Spending energy on one activity means foregoing another, so consider all the options — including cutting back on some of your grooming tasks.

Who could help you? Many personal care chores cannot be delegated; but you might ask your spouse or children to help lay out your clothes and equipment for the next day.

Ever since my son was quite young, he has watched and helped me with my medical regimen. It's a big help having him fetch the supplies; but more than that it has made him very comfortable with "Mommy's medicine stuff." I think it's good for kids — and husbands! — to get used to the equipment so it doesn't seem scary or strange.

How could your routine be modified to save energy? There are general principles and specific tips which can make your tasks less tiring. The first concerns positioning.

NEVER STAND WHEN YOU CAN SIT

The first way to save energy (your energy) on personal care tasks is to sit down. For this reason a bath is preferable to a shower; however a shower seat addresses the same principle. Sturdy, safe seats for the shower are available through mail-order catalogs and medical equipment suppliers. A hand-held shower head may be helpful in either case. It can eliminate some of the need to keep your arms raised overhead. You may prefer, at least sometimes, to sponge bathe at the sink. Put a chair or stool by the sink so you can sit there also.

SET-UP IS THE KEY TO EASE

You will save energy in the bath if you can avoid as much reaching, bending, and stretching as possible. Prepare your supplies before you bathe. Put a towel and robe within easy reach. Use something like a plastic bath caddy or bucket to hold all your toiletries: soap, shampoo, wash cloth, razor. It makes it easier to transport them from shower to sink. When you shop, look for products that make bathing easier such as liquid soaps, long-handled brushes, or shampoos which combine cleaning and conditioning.

When you bathe, begin by washing your hair because that takes the most energy. While in the bath or shower, you may want to shave, using either a disposable razor or a wet/dry electric razor. A stainless steel mirror can be mounted on the wall of the tub enclosure or on a telescoping arm to allow you to see what you are doing.

After you bathe, wrap in a big towel — or better still in a terry cloth robe — and sit down for a moment before you tackle your other chores.

Sitting by the basin you can shave or apply make-up. (You may need a tabletop mirror for this.) Try brushing your teeth while you are sitting down also. An electric toothbrush saves energy and there are many new inexpensive styles. If denture care is part of your routine, it can be set up on the sink counter the night before, as can medical dressings, ready to go in the morning.

The most effective way to save energy on grooming your hair is to choose a carefree style. Try to avoid a style that requires you to hold a blow dryer overhead every morning or to wind up rollers every night. Ask a hairdresser for advice on an easy wash-and-go style. Then all you will need is to brush or comb each morning and that can be done sitting down.

KEEP AHEAD OF HOUSEKEEPING

We recommend that you keep a sponge at the bathroom sink and make a habit of using it each morning. Before you stand up, take a quick swipe around the sink. A daily rinse and wipe will prevent a messy build-up of soap scum, toothpaste, and hair that could require heavy cleaning and scrubbing. In this case you are adding a small chore now to avoid a big, energy-consuming one later.

You can spare yourself another scrubbing chore by rinsing down the shower stall or tub each time you use it. Before you get out, use the hand-held shower head to hose down the walls, shower curtain and floor.

When you are ready to get dressed, sit down and reach for the clothes that you laid out earlier. More exertion is required to dress your lower body, so begin there.

CHOOSE A WARDROBE
TO FIT YOUR ENERGY BUDGET

As you become more aware of which tasks require extra energy, you will look at your wardrobe more critically. The following are tips that we've gathered from friends, clients, and our own experience.

Loose fitting clothes are easier to get on.

Elastic waists are preferable to snaps and zippers.

Panty hose are a struggle. Knee high or thigh high stockings are easier.

There are stocking and sock aides available, nifty little contraptions of various designs, which hold your stocking or sock open while you put your toe in and then assist you in pulling it up without bending.

Comfortable shoes save you energy all day long!

Long handled shoe horns save bending.

Dresses that fasten in the back are awkward.

Pullover shirts require extra energy because of the overhead work involved. Button fronts are better.

Brassieres with back closures are also difficult. You can opt for front closure styles or try fastening the bra in front and twisting to the back.

Boxer shorts are easier to don than jockey shorts.

Permanent press fabrics stay neat with little care.

Sweaters of acrylic yarn can be washed and dried with other laundry and save on hand-washing or trips to the dry cleaner.

VELCRO™ closures are really easy.

Dressing sticks are inexpensive and handy. They are sticks with a hook at the end you can use to pick up clothes from the floor, to pull on pants without bending, and to snag the other sleeve of a cardigan behind your back.

After you dress, take a breather. Plunging ahead with the day can cause events to snowball; so after your A.M. shuffle, relax. This does not have to mean inactivity. You can relax with your favorite morning beverage, prepared the night before in a thermos at your bedside. Listen to a radio or television newscast; jot down the day's plans on a pad kept by a comfortable chair or the bed; do needlework; read; practice relaxation techniques; think; have a quiet time with a loved one. The key is conserving that energy which is uniquely you, before continuing to meet the day.

Jaws: Conquering The Kitchen — 2

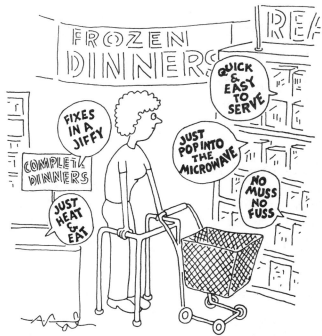

DELEGATION IS A KEY TO CONSERVING ENERGY

PLANNING CAN SAVE ENERGY

SIT TO WORK WHENEVER POSSIBLE

ORGANIZING SPACE IS A KEY TO CONSERVING ENERGY

MEAL PREPARATION

The kitchen is one room in the house that has been mightily affected by the advances of technology. Electrical appliances can do everything from open cans to wash dishes. Microwave ovens cook meals in minutes that would take hours in conventional ovens. It is not our intention in this chapter to recommend that you spend a lot of money on appliances. There is no denying, however, that if you can afford them, there are many kitchen gadgets available today which are real energy savers — *your* energy. Perhaps you can budget your money or make a wish list for gift givers in order to upgrade your kitchen in the future. We will discuss in this chapter things you can start doing today to conserve energy in traditional food preparation techniques.

Before you begin any task that requires a big expenditure of energy — and certainly cooking does — ask yourself, "Who should do this?"

DELEGATION IS A KEY TO CONSERVING ENERGY

Perhaps you are not the one who should prepare this meal. Your children, spouse, or roommate may be better candidates. You may find that rather than making all the meals yourself, a better role for you is supervising others in the kitchen or teaching someone else how to cook.

Another way to delegate this responsibility is to arrange for meals-on-wheels. In many communities this service provides a complete hot meal delivered at midday.

You can use more prepared foods — foods that someone else has prepared for you. For instance, many grocery stores now have salad bars. Besides enjoying a fresh salad without the work, consider some other options. You could take home the cut vegetables to use in soup or stew, or to steam for a hot dish. In the meat department look for chicken that is already cut up and ground beef shaped in patties. Your market may even have a selection of hot foods and salads at the deli counter. Survey the array of frozen foods in your stores. Using convenience foods is a way of delegating some of the work of meal preparation to someone else.

In my supermarket the butcher will cut meats to my order and, when they are not busy, the deli counter staff will slice vegetables for me.

Take-out food is another idea. We do not recommend the traditional "fast foods" which are fried and salty. But restaurants, like the supermarkets, are finding a growing market among busy, health conscious singles and working parents for ready-to-go foods. You can benefit from this trend. Many fine restaurants now offer a take-out menu.

PLANNING IS A KEY TO CONSERVING ENERGY

If you have determined that it is best for you to prepare a meal, then it is time for planning. By thinking through what you are going to do before you do it, your work becomes more efficient. You use your energy wisely and not wastefully.

Plot out your menus for the next few days. It may help to write them down. Look over your meal plans for cooking tasks that can be combined. For instance when you are soft boiling an egg for Monday's breakfast, hard boil another one for Wednesday's egg salad sandwich. While you are brewing a cup of coffee or tea in the morning, you could make a pot to rewarm later, fill a thermos, or make a pitcher of iced tea or coffee. If you are paring and slicing vegetables for a salad tonight, do extras for later in the week.

Many recipes lend themselves to making ahead. So when you do devote some energy to cooking, double your recipe and freeze the extra. Another day will come when you will appreciate having something that just needs to be reheated. Freeze breads and muffins and take them out as you use them. When you need to chop half an onion or dice half a pepper for a recipe, do the whole thing and freeze the extra. In fact you can freeze anything as long as it does not have mayonnaise in it — and we have!

A wonderful shower gift for a new mother, or a welcome home gift for someone just discharged from the hospital, is a cooler filled with frozen dinners for the freezer. Each friend makes his or her own specialty. It's personal and very practical, too. (Be sure to check on any dietary restrictions or allergies.)

There are a number of cookbooks out now that specialize in fast, easy recipes. Check the library or bookstore.

Each time you reach to open a cupboard, each time you bend to get a utensil from a drawer, each time you pull open the refrigerator door you use energy. Those little bits of expended energy add up to make cooking a fatiguing activity. Before you start, think about everything you will need to do. Try to open the cupboard, the drawer, and the refrigerator only once each. Gather all your ingredients and equipment before you begin. Avoid as much of the reaching and bending as possible by planning ahead.

"Reachers" are long handled tools that may be helpful in your household. They come in many styles with a variety of grips.

A wheeled cart is very handy to have in the kitchen. You can use it to transport things. It can help eliminate extra trips between the refrigerator and workspace and it is easier to push a cart than to carry everything. Use it to set the table in one trip and clear the dishes later. It can take pots for you from the sink to the stove. The cart should be tall enough so you are not always bending over it. If you use a cane or walker, a cart on casters is important for your safety. Use your cane or walker for support and let your body nudge the cart along as you go. Do not use the cart in place of your walking aid. If you use a wheelchair, a cart may be handy to pull beside you.

A wheeled cart is not the only way to carry things in the kitchen. Big pockets in a smock or apron can take small items. A large basket or caddy allows you to carry items while leaving the other hand free for a cane. There are also trays designed to attach to walkers and wheel-chairs.

SIT TO WORK WHENEVER POSSIBLE

The most important piece of advice we can give you in this chapter (and you will find it in other chapters too!) is to sit down. Therefore, the most important item for conserving your energy in the kitchen is a stool or chair. If you have a kitchen table, you could do your meal preparation there. If you have a stool or high chair you could work at the countertop. A swivel chair, such as the barstool style, may be convenient for you. Many have a footrest bar, but if not you will want a footstool of some kind for support. A chair you already have can be raised by adding leg extenders. Chair leg extenders come with and without casters and are easily attached by tightening wing nuts.

You will find it easier to sit at the counter if you have the door removed from a base cabinet to make some leg room. You could clear room for your legs under the sink too in order to wash dishes sitting down. If you must stand at the sink, put down a small rug. You will be surprised at what a difference a little cushioning can make.

Some sinks are quite deep so you may find that whether you sit or stand, the bottom is an uncomfortable stretch away. The solution may simply be to place a dishpan on an upturned pot in the bottom of the sink.

Adjust the height of the chair or work surface until you find the most comfortable position. You want to be able to sit with good posture and to avoid bending over your work. The ingredients and equipment you have gathered should be arranged in a semicircle within your normal reach.

There are some techniques to simplify the cooking itself. Adapt your favorite recipes to cut out unnecessary steps. Try to use "one bowl" or "one pot" methods as much as possible. A rubber mat, suction cups, or a nonskid pad will hold a mixing bowl steady so you don't have to. Slide rather than lift your equipment, such as pots from the sink to the range. Whenever possible let gravity do the work. Put a pan in your lap below the level of the cutting board and push the vegetables into it.

ORGANIZING SPACE IS A KEY TO CONSERVING ENERGY

As you become more conscious of the energy costs of your routine cooking tasks, you will recognize that there are changes you should make in the organization of your kitchen workspace. Foods and equipment that you use most often should be stored where they are most accessible — or not stored at all. Anything you use every day is probably best left out on the counter. Watch yourself as you prepare a meal. Are there some things you reach for repeatedly? They should be kept right at hand. Are there items on the prime shelves, the ones that are easiest for you to reach, which you rarely use? They should be stored elsewhere to free up that space.

The organization of the kitchen in each household is very idiosyncratic. We offer some arrangements that work for us to help you start thinking about simple changes you could make in your own kitchen.

During our long New England winters we keep the tea kettle filled with water on the back burner of the range all the time. Our cocoa, tea, and coffee are in the cabinet right beside it.

Utensils we use often stay on the counter next to the stove in a pretty, old stoneware pitcher with a chipped spout.

I like to bake, but don't do it often so my baking supplies are in the harder-to-reach corner cupboard. When I do bake, everything is there together: flour, honey, baking powder, raisins, cookie cutters.

My grandmother's new refrigerator had a lot of low shelf space that was hard for her to see and reach, so my father built a wooden base and raised the whole thing up six inches.

Lazy Susans can improve access to the items in a cupboard, the refrigerator, or in the corner of the countertop. A lazy Susan in the center of the table can bring the foods to you without a stretch. There are other ways to make the most of your storage space: swing-out shelves for cans and jars, pull-out racks for pots and pans, and stacking storage bins for vegetables. There are shallow shelf units that attach to the inside of a cabinet door for extra storage within easy reach. Magnetic or suction hooks can hold potholders, measuring spoons, or recipes. All of these items are readily available at hardware and discount stores and by mail order.

It is annoying to waste a lot of effort struggling to open a container. Look for brands that come in easy-to-manage packaging and transfer foods to containers that you can handle. There are a variety of devices you can buy to help open jars. Some are designed to mount on the wall and fold flat when not in use. There are combination jar and can openers and there are gadgets which can handle the push-and-turn childproof caps.

When it is time to clean up, ask again, "Who should do this?" Delegation is the best way to spare your energy; but organization and planning can make the work easier.

Soaking dishes saves on scrubbing; so when you finish cooking slide the dirty pots over to the sink and fill them with warm soapy water. After you eat you can put the dishes in to soak too and then sit down for a breather. The dishes will be easier to wash and you will have more stamina after a few minutes rest.

When you wash the dishes, leave them to air dry in a drainboard. Before you leave the sink, wipe it clean and, sponge still in hand, wipe up any spills on the range or counter. It is a good idea to keep some cleanser right at the sink and make this quick swipe cleaning a routine. A build-up of dried spills requires the kind of heavy scouring you want to avoid.

When the dishes are dry, set the table for the next meal right from the drainboard or dishwasher. It is inefficient to put dishes away in the cupboard only to get them out again a little while later.

Frequent light housecleaning is less taxing than heavy cleaning; so store the equipment you need to clean the kitchen in the kitchen and use it briefly but often.

I keep a small laundry bag in the kitchen for dishtowels and table linens.

Take advantage of the variety of disposable dinnerware available. When you are having company and know you will be spending extra energy on cooking and socializing, use paper plates and cups to save energy on the clean-up.

Good nutrition is essential to our health and well-being. We cannot let our fear of "Jaws" lurking in the kitchen keep us out of the water. Delegate as much of the meal preparation as possible. Organize the kitchen space and plan the work so your energy is used effectively. Sit down when you can and keep ahead of the cleaning. Hopefully these tips will help you navigate the shark infested waters of the kitchen and reach a tasty, healthy diet on the far shore.

Traffic Control — 3

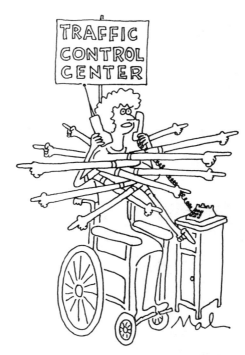

DAYS FOR ERRANDS
GROUP ERRANDS GEOGRAPHICALLY
FIND AND USE DELIVERY SERVICES
THE TELEPHONE IS MAN'S BEST FRIEND
USE CARRYING AIDS

ERRANDS AND
HOUSEHOLD MANAGEMENT

Daily life can mirror an officer attempting to control the ebb and flow of traffic at a busy intersection. Upon rising each morning we are very much officers directing the flow of endless errands and household tasks. There is the shopping, yard work, laundry, appointments, chauffeuring, banking and the dreaded "unexpecteds."

Chapter One talked about energy conservation in personal care and Chapter Two brought us into the kitchen. In Traffic Control we will focus on efficiently executing the various tasks and household management skills encountered day-to-day. This is imperative in order to optimize your energy. Visualize your days first in terms of a month, then a week and then a day. Jot down a list of known appointments and errands at the beginning of each month on a large calendar. This can include physician appointments, get-togethers, dry cleaners, haircuts, beauty parlor appointments, children's activities, market days and so on. Remember to put the phone numbers down as well, thus saving the proverbial hunt.

The last evening of the month I begin my next month's thinking. I wait until everyone is quieted for the night, put on a record and start to plan. Already on my calendar, in red ink, are birthdays and anniversaries I want to remember. Yearly I transfer this information from calendar-to-calendar, with appropriate additions and deletions. Every other entry on the calendar is done in pencil for easy erasure.

I have a paperweight on my desk for the sole purpose

of leaving notes about various appointments or errands. Everyone knows that if they do not leave their appointment information or requests here, it will not be put on the calendar and probably will be forgotten!

The best size and style calendar is a large desk pad calendar. There are very big squares to write in and you are able to sit while planning and juggling. If you do not have the desk or table space, these calendars can be hung. They are available through most large department or discount stores, as well as through stationery supply stores, stationery supply catalogs and larger pharmacies. More specialized, erasable wall calendars are also available through the supply catalogs and stationers, however, they are definitely more costly.

DESIGNATE DAYS FOR ERRANDS

Certain days are best designated for certain tasks, so try and arrange other appointments and errands around these. Marketing is best done on a day that will guarantee greatest item availability and freshness. Beauty parlors and barbers are usually closed on a certain day each week, so plan accordingly. Many after-school activities are scheduled ahead on specific days. Try to accomplish at-home tasks, such as laundry, on these days to decrease the number of trips you make.

You will be surprised at how much energy you save yourself. By creating this monthly framework, your weekly and daily planning will be easier and energy efficient. At the beginning of each week, check to see if all appointments have been written down and then fill in those special or extra tasks that have popped up. Always try and fit these in and around your monthly designated task days. I keep a post-it note pad by my calendar. At the beginning of the week each family member gets a list of their appointments or tasks stuck to their bureau. No more "you didn't remind me" chorus in our house.

GROUP ERRANDS GEOGRAPHICALLY

Daily planning takes into account many factors and the best possible way to conserve energy is to group errands geographically. Make a list each day of all activities and then arrange them so that the most efficient use of your time and rest is made. Circular patterns of travel are best. List everywhere you must go and then plan your travel accordingly. First locate the destinations furthest from you and set your circular pattern to get there. For example, if you must drop off clothes at the dry cleaner, do banking, return books to the library and go to the market — start by identifying the furthest location and begin and end with home. Your route should be planned so that entering and leaving the various stops along the way will go with the flow of traffic, instead of against it. Taking a right into traffic instead of taking a left and having to cut across traffic lanes, will accomplish this.

Some of your stops will be on the way to the furthest location, and some on return from the furthest location. I searched a long time to find a community with easy access to almost all my needs and drew a sketch of the town and surrounding areas so when planning my errands I could establish my route at a glance. This also helped me teach my son the value of maps.

If you must travel a great distance for an appointment or errand, make it the only task for the day to decrease exhaustion. If you can combine the longer trip with a relaxing visit at a friend's or a leisurely lunch break, you will rejuvenate yourself for the return leg of your journey.

FIND AND USE DELIVERY SERVICES

Making use of delivery services can appear costly. However, they can actually be more cost effective in terms of your health and energy reserves. What you spend in dollars is gained in your ability to be more productive for a longer period of time during the day. As the popularity for delivery services increases, the cost will go down. You can save these services for days when you just physically or emotionally cannot manage a trip.

Check out the phone directory yellow pages and community bulletin boards for services offered. Your local newspaper will also have a section in the classifieds. Most smaller markets offer delivery of groceries for either a flat rate or per mile. By creating a routine, "stock" list of frequently used items, the bulk of your marketing can be done from your home.

Milkmen still provide door-to-door service in many communities. They carry all types of dairy products, as well as breads and fruit juices.

Many pizzerias and smaller restaurants will deliver.

Senior centers offer meals-on-wheels, as well as some churches and synagogues.

Cleaners are beginning to offer pick-up and delivery

services, especially in larger cities and their surrounding communities.

There are new and expanding services that will run errands and market for you.

Teenagers and college students are looking for ways to earn extra money and are willing to provide assistance on a routine basis. Contact your local high school guidance office and college student affairs office for names.

THE TELEPHONE IS MAN'S BEST FRIEND

Having spent a great deal of time running to places, only to find that they were closed or did not have the item I wanted, taught me the value of the telephone. So many tasks can be accomplished efficiently and with virtually no exertion by calling ahead. Shopping can also be done by phone and most catalogs have 800 numbers (toll free) with door-to-door delivery. Always inquire about ordering and delivery options for all your needs.

Many manufacturers extend mail order services, at discount prices, for their merchandise. Always get the name, number and address of an item's manufacturer and contact them. .

Do not let a store's response of "no delivery or phone orders" deter you. Ask to speak to the manager and explain your needs. Most stores will find some way to assist.

Be willing to do business with another place if delivery and ordering are services they offer.

DO NOT DO BULK BUYING ON YOUR OWN

Cargo carrying can be a great energy sapper and physical debilitator. If you have the tendency to be a beast-of-burden, stop! You should never do bulk buying on your own. Try to intersperse purchasing different items throughout the month instead of in one trip. Remember, everything loaded must be unloaded.

Marketing is notorious for bulk buying. If you can, use delivery services and break your shopping list down into what we call P.M.S. (Planned Meal Shopping). Not only will the cargo load be lighter, but you will spend less time actually marketing.

P.M.S. is marketing each week according to a five or seven day menu plan. This decreases impulse buying, saves money and definitely lessens the baggage load. Ask the baggers to pack the bags lightly, with perishable items separate from the rest. If not offered, ask for assistance carrying the bags to your vehicle and loading them. If you must bulk-buy, or shop at a food warehouse where no bagging or carrying services are offered, take a friend or family member with you. P.M.S. was a surprise success in our home. Not only did it afford me the chance to eradicate bulk buying, but our diet became healthier. By thinking about specific needs for meals over an entire week, I was able to plan balanced menus and increase the varieties of offerings. Everyone got into the swing by choosing a meal they enjoyed most or helped with ideas for accompaniments to my choices for main courses.

My son's interest burgeoned into a desire to cook for himself and we spend companionable times each week cooking together. He now has confidence in his ability to provide for himself. No fast-or-prepared food anymore! The right food purchases and nutritious, tasty and easy-to-prepare meals and snacks are now readily available.

USE CARRYING AIDS

It is indeed heartening to see many markets and stores providing motorized shopping vehicles for their customers. This is a definite boon for those physically impaired or with poor energy reserves. If these are not available, portable and collapsible wheeled utility carts can be purchased fairly inexpensively. These are either pushed or pulled and provide just the right amount of cargo-carrying space for optimum energy expenditure. A child's red-wagon can be used to trundle items.

Collapsible, electric transportation carts can be purchased or leased. They fold into your trunk, but are costly and heavy to manage on your own. This could be a long-term, planned purchase item or one for your holiday wish list.

A homemade dumb waiter can assist in cargo carrying at home. The principle is the same as that of a pulley clothesline, only set at an angle for transporting items at either a slant or up and down. You place your cargo in the attached box or canvas bag and pull. The pulley lets you pull with greater ease than carrying bundles up or down.

A baby carriage or stroller is easily pushed and special cargo carriers are designed for wheelchairs and walkers.

DELEGATE TASKS

A tenet of true energy conservation is assigning certain chores and tasks to others in order to maintain a healthy and happy quality of life. This is called delegating. When first thinking about this you may tend to shy away from delegation in light of achieving independence. By learning to creatively delegate you will find a greater independence because there is leftover energy to do more.

A variation on the barter system is to arrange "help-visiting" with friends. By allowing your friends to assist in chores or tasks requiring great energy output, you can have an enjoyable visit while accomplishing something difficult for you. The "help-visiting" idea has provided my family with a now-and-then break in tasks necessarily delegated to them. It frees their time and I get to visit with my friends.

Sometimes delegating a task can be as simple as preparation of lunch with an invited guest. Do not hesitate to include your guests in the putting together of a meal. Companionable meal preparation extends your time for visiting and can be great fun. Exhausting yourself in the kitchen, while friends sit waiting, will only create an uncomfortable time for all. You will not be able to fully enjoy your visit or meal and your guests will be uncomfortable if they notice — or find out later — that you "tuckered" yourself out because of them.

If you can do a particular task or chore that a friend may not like, try mutually exchanging this for something you need to have done. Through this exchange of services both benefit. If it can be combined with sharing each other's company, so much the better. Enjoying a task actually lessens the energy spent in doing it, for our emotions can be energy "sappers" as well as enhancers.

Composing letters and notes has always been a dreaded task for my mother and hemming is difficult for me to manage physically. We have come up with a system where I compose various letters for her, while she hems an article of clothing for me. We share a cup of tea or coffee and catch up on our news.

Proof-reading and typing manuscripts is both enjoyable and possible for me to do. My college roommate could not type, so we swapped chores. She ran up and down the dorm stairs to do my laundry and I typed her term papers.

A friend of ours has swapped the chore of baking two dozen muffins for her neighbor in exchange for the weekly marketing. While her neighbor unpacks the groceries, she puts on a pot of coffee for them to share and enjoy together.

Most people want to feel good about themselves and to aid and assist others whenever possible. Helping others is a component of building self-esteem. When you afford someone the chance to do something for you through delegation of tasks, a sense of well-being and pride can result. It is important to realize that true friendship and family is the ability and opportunity to give and take. You do yourself and those around you a disservice if you do not learn to ask for help.

My son had his chores to do around the house, but nothing very difficult, because I felt the household tasks were my responsibility. Once, when I was hospitalized, he overheard someone say I was doing much-too-much of the physical household chores such as vacuuming, trash, garage sweeping and moving around furniture. He said, crying, that he could take care of me and he would do everything. I reassured him that it was not his role to take care of me, but mine to take care of him. I also promised to let him do more, but not everything. By keeping this promise I found that he swelled with pride when he could boast about helping his mom and no guilt resulted when I became ill. He found he could rise to a challenge and learned to think problems through. His self-esteem definitely improved. I also learned to share my hidden, physical realities with him, dispelling any misconceptions or pity. I was a mom but we could do things together.

PUNCTUATE EACH DAY WITH RESTS

Balancing the tasks of life with periods of rest are so essential to those with depleted energy reserves. Planning rest periods daily are vital to maintaining a modicum of the status quo. It is a practiced art. First you must actually convince yourself it is necessary. Think back to a day when you did not stop for a minute and remember how you felt by the end of the day and the day after. For anyone with low energy, this generally spells disaster. Rest can come in a variety of ways, so try not to think that total withdrawal from activities is necessary all the time. Your rest periods can really be simple breathers.

A favorite get-away for me is the wing chair in my bedroom. I have the ability to close my door and put on the noon news for half-an-hour. If I choose, I eat a light lunch here as well.

The use of a telephone answering machine is fantastic for taking a break. Get into the habit of choosing a break time from the phone. No calls will be missed.

When driving to and from errands, pull over to the side of the road, or in a parking lot, and close your eyes for a few moments.

Stopping for a refreshing or warming beverage between errands and household chores will provide respite.

Take that coffee break and do not work through it.

Visualization and relaxation techniques can be mastered and used in almost any situation.

Clue your family and friends into your need for rest periods. Children can understand quiet times, and can even learn to share in them — if it is the routine.

Before or after meal preparation, take five minutes to rejuvenate yourself.

Naps in mid-afternoon can give that extra boost for the remainder of the day.

Rest periods may be flexible to permit change at the last moment. Many factors can influence plans, such as harsh weather, medical problems, fatigue or pain. All of these are great energy depleters. Awareness of the pitfalls will help in your overall planning.

Weather is a force to be reckoned with and for the person with low energy, it can be devastating. During a three day period a few years ago, I did not allow myself any relaxation breaks. I did not listen to the weather forecast even though it was mid-winter in New England and merrily set out for an errand about forty-five minutes away. Before I completed my errand, the snow

30

started to fall heavily and roads became treacherous. I had to stop frequently and scrape ice from the windshield and the driving was extremely tense. I reached home dangerously exhausted. It put me out of commission for two days — two days that could have been productive.

DO ADVANCE WORK FOR EMERGENCIES

No matter how well organized you are, the unexpected is bound to occur and emergencies can compound themselves. Doing advance work for emergencies will greatly enhance your ability to function with optimum energy and can prevent further complications. When mapping out a route for travel, make sure you can easily summon aid. Car phones are terrific but unaffordable to most. In lieu of this, you can do many things to assure assistance on the road and in emergencies.

Plan your route to be traveled. City streets may be slower and more congested than isolated roads, but if you are alone, they will afford you access to phones and alternate modes of transportation.

If you plan on doing many errands or traveling a long distance, another driver can assist by relieving you before you get fatigued. In an emergency situation, having another person along can be of supreme importance.

Carry pertinent emergency, medical, insurance and historical information with you at all times. A manila folder is perfect. Your documents are kept neat and safe.

A canteen or thermos of water is great for either vehicle or passenger use. Crackers or dry cereal in a zip-lock bag will assure some nourishment.

Carry flares in case of emergency and have your vehicle serviced regularly.

Every other time you fill your gas tank, check your vehicle fluids and tire pressure. Make sure your spare is in good condition.

Carry a change of clothes, basic toiletries, medical dressing supplies and medicines in a satchel kept in the trunk.

A roll of paper towels comes in handy for windshields and spills.

A telephone credit card will provide you with access to a pay phone.

Motorist aid boxes are frequently found on major interstates. Learn how to use them by contacting your local state police.

A major credit card can provide you with payment for an unexpected motel stay or medical intervention.

In the home, situations requiring aid can happen frequently. Being prepared for emergencies will greatly reduce the anxiety and stress. Make sure you can access phones or emergency buttons easily and from a variety of locations. Plan with a neighbor or friend to have you call at a certain time each day and let at least two people know where you keep a house key outside — or provide them with one. Emergency phone numbers should be close at hand and with programmable phones, you can simply push a button. Teaching young and old to dial or go for help in an emergency is definitely valuable.

On the market are alert call systems. The idea is excellent, but be sure to thoroughly investigate the cost, hidden costs, merchandise durability and warranty. Your local and state public health departments can provide you with reliable information regarding these items, as well as state departments of consumer protection.

A young patient of mine woke one morning with chills, vomiting and a high fever due to septicemia. She rolled over and pushed her neighbor's button on her programmable phone. She was unable to get to the door due to extreme weakness, so she was lucky she had given her neighbor a key to let herself in. The neighbor phoned the doctor, got her to the hospital and took care of her cats while she was hospitalized. It was less stressful to be able to phone a friend and be reassured that her home and pets would be taken care of, than to call an ambulance. Preparation paid off.

Errands and household tasks can become manageable and energy efficient. Emergencies can be prepared for and stress reduced. Just have a bit of perseverance, be flexible, think and plan ahead, and make sure you build in plenty of time for rest. The rewards will show in the smooth ebb and flow of your life's daily traffic patterns.

Olympic
High Hurdles — 4

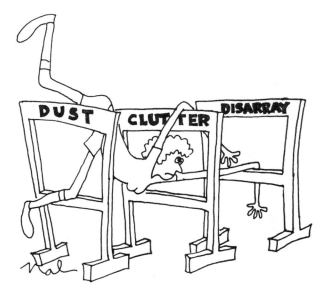

HUMOR CAN GO A LONG WAY

UNCLUTTER AND REDIRECT TRAFFIC

**DESIGNATE A ROOM ACCORDING TO USAGE,
NOT CONVENTION**

LANDSCAPE FOR LOW MAINTENANCE

**LIVING WITH OTHERS CAN LEAD TO
GREATER INDEPENDENCE**

STAIRS AND ARCHITECTURE

Home is where the heart is.
Home sweet home.
Home's haven.
Home at last ...

How wonderful if these colloquialisms were true! More often than not, we look around our home and sigh. The dust, clutter and disarray are repetitive hurdles and if you have the problem of low energy, these hurdles can appear insurmountable. But take heart, for there are ways to creatively structure, re-structure, streamline and control your home's style for energy efficiency — your energy efficiency. Not all will be practical to do, but the idea can be manipulated to fit your particular circumstance and situation.

HUMOR CAN GO A LONG WAY

By finding the humor in a situation you can do much to alleviate the tensions and pressures that come with taking care of a home, no matter what the size.

A feisty young woman had a cross-stitch sampler hanging by her front door that said "You certainly can't eat off my floor, but then again, nothing's going to bite your ankles either." She felt that anyone entering would get a laugh and at the same time she never felt like apologizing if things were not quite up-to-snuff.

An elderly neighbor would cut out quips from magazines or newspapers pertaining to household chores. By putting them on her refrigerator she would be reminded that things really were not too bad and that others were experiencing similar hassles.

CONTROL ACCESS

It might be surprising, but you can begin energy conservation at your entrances. Entrances are doors into the home. People, pets, insects, dirt, dust, mud and wet gravitate toward these doors, so start by controlling access to them and master where and how you enter.

Using one or two entrances confines clutter and mess. One entry can be for guests or delivery and one for family traffic. Mats on both sides of the door are terrific work savers and should be long enough to handle the job. Extra dollars spent on quality mats will provide a durable product and save cleaning time and energy.

A broom-finished (rough) concrete sidewalk or ramp leading to a covered entryway helps eliminate dirt, mud and wet *before* entering. Steps contribute to the accumulation of dirt and it takes work to keep them dirt and sand free. The flooring of the inside entrance is best if made of heavy vinyl, quarry tile or natural stone. The less grooves or indentations there are the better.

The walls of entries can be energy savers as well. If the surfaces are smooth instead of textured, flying dirt can't settle and it is easier to wipe down. Semigloss enamel paint, panelling and vinyl wallpaper are a few examples of energy-efficient materials.

Closets at entrances collect flying dust and dirt. They also become miscellaneous storage compartments. The best arrangement is a small closet at the guest entrance

and a coat rack, shelf and boot mat at the family entry.
By eliminating a closet at the frequented door, you eliminate the tendency to store clutter.

CREATE GUIDANCE CENTERS

Guidance centers operate much like a symphony con-
ductor standing on the podium. He orchestrates what
happens on a vast stage from his strategic position. In
the home, your guidance centers coordinate and direct
activities, help concentrate cleaning and make space
work to your advantage. Frequented entries are where
you can first use the idea of a guidance center.

My home incorporates the idea of a satellite guidance
center in its family entry. When we come through the
door from the garage, there is a plastic storage bin to the
left of the stairs. It contains a small trash receptacle,
kleenex, towel and broom. When the time is right, we
add seasonal paraphernalia. The rule of the roost is to
empty those coat pockets before entering the house and
to wipe your greasy or dirty hands with the towel. When
noses are running, no one races upstairs from the outside to get a kleenex, tracking in mud and dirt. It is
ready and waiting to be used and discarded right at the
entry. Especially dear to my heart is the ability for everyone to brush off shoe dirt, or pesky leaves or snow
from an overcoat. To the right of the stairs are hooks for
coats, a shelf for hats and mittens and a boot-mate mat.
Everyone knows what I want and where I want it done
when they enter my house!

When designing the main guidance center of a house,
evaluate where you spend the most time using varied

38

items to organize and enjoy daily living. Satellite centers, such as the one in the family entry-way, offer less varied usage and are more specific in nature. The main guidance center is your command post.

A must for the main guidance center is a comfortable chair with good support, a footstool and good lighting. Keep the telephone, calendar and writing materials within easy reach so you can plan, schedule and chat in comfort. Relaxation is just as important, so keep near a TV or radio, magazines, books and hobby materials. You will find time is maximized with little effort in a well-planned, main guidance center. Traffic, work, play and confusion become organized soldiers with few skirmishes.

Our home has a strategically located study, which acts as the main guidance center. Everyone can be seen or heard when they enter through the guest and family entrances or from above. There is no chance to escape detection. My family fondly calls this main guidance center "the command post!" All wall space is used for perimeter placement of furniture, which includes three desks, a file cabinet, and bookcase. The central, open floor space that results from perimeter furniture placement makes cleaning a lot easier. The addition of casters to the swivel chairs allow easy movement from desk to desk.

My "post chair" is at my correspondence desk, where many coordinating and information items are located. There is a large, calendar desk pad with more than adequate space to write in activities, events and for noting special days. The desk pad calendar is more energy efficient because I can sit to look or write, rather than stand

and reach up to use a wall calendar. The telephone has programmable capacity for ease in dialing and an extra long cord for mobility. Our answering machine is great when I am out and also for when I am just too tired to deal with any interruptions. A handy plastic coated, wire basket for my keys and handicap placard mean I always know where these items are. Energy is not wasted for the proverbial key hunt. A pencil holder and rolodex phone/address card file are within easy reach and my bills are directly in front of me in a pretty painted container. There is no confusion when they have to be located and paid! Various stationery and desk items are located in the drawer for easy access.

A pretty array of baskets are on the wall in front of the post desk and double as mail and message holders. To the right is a cork board for those all-important schedules and notes, and two plastic storage crates are turned on their sides on the floor below this. They double as extra bookshelves for reference books and files — no bending required.

A wonderful old rocking chair with an heirloom footstool allows for relaxation and is easily accessible to my command post, should the need arise. My combination record player, cassette player and radio are located on the large bookshelf and my embroidery bag lies close at hand. My father's favorite saying when he views me directing family flow is "little Caesar at work sitting!"

Locating a satellite control center in your bedroom can be that no-cost getaway you have been looking for — no cost to the pocket or to your energy. We have found that by having a phone, clock-radio, pad and pencil placed at the bedside, you can maintain the coordination and flow of household activities. If there is room, a small chair by the bed will afford visitors and family members a place to join you in relaxation.

UNCLUTTER AND REDIRECT TRAFFIC

It is surprisingly easy to create living space that will decrease work. If you don't want everyone emptying their pockets onto the lamp table by the door — get rid of the table. If you do not want loitering in a particular area, relocate or eliminate a chair.

An elderly neighbor gave me her rule for decorating: "If there is a seat, someone will sit on it; if there is a table, something will be put on it; and if it is in the way, you will go around."

Use a chair, sofa, table or wall to redirect traffic flow around an area you want kept clear. It is remarkable how tracked-in dirt, mess and clutter disappear, or are confined, when employing these simple tricks. Cleaning is easier too!

Home should be the place to escape from stress and discomfort, especially if you are dealing with low energy. Surrounding yourself with low maintenance furniture, materials and decor leads to enjoyment. Try to strike a balance between your taste and practicality.

CLEAN WITH ENERGY CONSERVATION IN MIND

Cleaning is work and one of the leading causes of stress and exhaustion. It is important to classify your household contents and decor by equating them with the degree of maintenance required. If you recondition

41

yourself to view cleaning chores as groups of items requiring daily, frequent or infrequent cleaning, your energy will be saved and time gained. It is OK to learn to live with more dirt temporarily, if the gain is feeling relaxed and stronger because you budgeted your energy.

What constitutes a daily maintenance item, is of course, up to the individual. However, by thinking of repetitive daily activities you come up with an overview that includes:

eating tables
counters
stovetops
sinks
beds
trash

Frequent maintenance items can generally be classified as needing weekly care. There will be times, however, when they are not cleaned for a month or more! By attempting to do these items weekly you will save on the extra energy needed for scrubbing, versus simpler and lighter cleaning. These can include:

tubs
showers
toilets
dusting
entranceways
carpeted floors
floors (kitchen & bath)
the yard

The best-loved cleaning tasks are those you do not have to think about more than every couple of months — or annually! Some of these are:

exterior of house
windows
window coverings
closets
under and behind large appliances and furniture

No matter what the cleaning chore, always keep in mind that your health and leisure are priority issues. Perhaps your cleaning routines are not up to your old standards, but a healthier and happier you is definitely worth the change.

I can remember a warm summer day, sitting on my ottoman and crying as the sun brightly illuminated the bay window. The year's accumulation of dirt was so very visible. I just had not been able to clean the windows every six months or so as I usually did. My neighbor chose this inopportune time to visit. Seeing my reddened eyes she empathetically questioned the cause. When I told her, she actually laughed, saying, "Honey, you just have to learn that when the sun shines in you close the shades!"

UNIFORMITY AND SIMPLICITY
STREAMLINE UPKEEP

Upkeep requires tools and the more varied the surfaces you have, the more specialized cleaning tools you will need. Keep to the tenets of simplicity and uniformity and you will find cleaning routines and equipment are streamlined. There is less work.

A disabled woman offered the wonderful hint that "three is the key to cleaning — broom, mop/cloth and vacuum." Walls, furniture, linoleum and carpet are terri-

43

tories for the vacuum. It dusts and cleans. What she calls a "mop/cloth" is a sponge mop with VELCRO™ attached dust rag secured to the handle. This takes care of floors needing a wash and tables needing a polish. A clean sweep with the broom eliminates dirt on the stoop and in the basement and garage.

Uniformity in furniture style and perimeter (wall) placement will greatly reduce maintenance, give an aura of spaciousness and aid in traffic control. By placing furniture along the wall space you can clean a greater area without moving anything. If you place a piece of furniture "in the way," people will redirect themselves to go around the obstacle, saving wear-and-tear and up-keep of an area you want avoided on a daily basis. Simple lines and camouflage techniques for upholstery and carpet create the illusion of cleanliness. You do not have to give up individual expression or style — only extra work!

Pattern and design in upholstery hide wear, tear and imperfections.

Sculptured, low-nap, medium colored, stain-resistant carpets are great at camouflaging dirt and wear.

Secured (stationary) couch cushions prevent scattering and you do not have to constantly straighten them.

Wood tables clean with ease and formica eating surfaces reduce clean-up time and increase durability.

The lighter the surface color and non-gloss, the less dirt shows.

When the floors and walls are uniform in color, it is easy to clean, repair and decorate. The expression of your personality can come through by creating decor with wall-hangings and accents.

Knick-knack clutter can be an energy sapper. Try to establish a single focus in a room and use the introduction of color and style to enhance simplicity. You do not have to discard those favorite treasures; merely keep a few out at a time and rotate them as frequently as you want.

Avoid the irresistible urge to put framed photographs on end tables, bookcases, bureaus and coffee tables. Hanging them eliminates the need to move them when dusting and picking them up when they fall.

Wicker mail baskets come in a variety of shapes, sizes and colors. They cost little and many can be purchased through mail-order houses. Place them near your frequented entry and double their value: a terrific wall treatment and you will not forget to mail those letters and bills.

Plants require care and energy to keep healthy. Consolidating them in one area and hanging as many as possible will make watering and care easier. Silk flower arrangements need a minimum of care and can be purchased fairly inexpensively. You can simplify even more by using floral and plant prints in your curtains, upholstery and wallcoverings.

The kitchen should contain items that are readily cleaned. If frills are you, put a pattern in your curtain, vinyl wallpaper, stencil, or floor covering. The kitchen is generally the hub of activities. You may want to locate your main guidance center in the kitchen, utilizing one section of the counter top, a drawer, the phone, calendar, message-board and comfortable kitchen chair.

Magnets on the refrigerator, if strong and of a good quality, can assist in keeping messages, lists and those all-important school papers in a central area. They are decorative as well.

Less-is-more is so important in the kitchen. Evaluate the function of each kitchen item by taking into consideration the number of people using it, food preferences, frequency of entertaining and formal or informal dining style. Also consider the volume of food for a given week, daily routines, traffic patterns, budget, personal preferences and essential accessories and appliances. This evaluation process will assist in uncluttering and reorganizing the kitchen.

Eliminate any item from within easy reach that must be thought about twice.

Infrequently used items should be stored on top shelves, in deep cabinets or discarded.

Bureaus should be uncluttered and, if at all possible, do not attach a mirror. Instead, locate a wall space on the back of a door for a full-length mirror. This will serve a variety of purposes, from grooming to dressing.

There is a burgeoning market for maximizing closet storage and efficiency, making the necessity of a bureau obsolete, save for aesthetic value. You can create shelving, drawer, and hanging storage space in your closet with a minimum of effort and cost. Local department or hardware stores carry such items, as well as catalogs, for at-home shopping and delivery.

Our family had a closet party one weekend. Everyone brought their own brown-bag lunch. By dinner, my bureau had been moved to my sister-in-law's van and my closet transformed into efficient space. I had more room to store my clothing and my sister-in-law now had a bureau. It was a great visiting and working weekend.

If you have children's bedrooms, you can maximize storage space and make cleaning easier. Stackable plastic crates and rolling carts of all sizes and for multiple uses are available in bright colors. If there is a plastic crate by their door for laundry, they can scoop it up every day and take it to the main laundry basket.

DESIGNATE A ROOM ACCORDING TO USAGE, NOT CONVENTION

If you frequently entertain formally, then a dining room is both aesthetic and practical. Try to keep the lines of the furniture simple and the table covered with a tablecloth when not in use. This reduces the need to dust and polish. When entertaining, place mats placed on top of the table cloth decrease the risk of staining the cloth itself and are much easier to clean. If storage of china and crystal is necessary due to frequent use, then opt for simplicity, once again, in a hutch or sideboard. Remember, the more you see the more you clean.

My main guidance center used to be my living room. I took a radical step and eliminated my dining room, turning it into my living room! Since I store better dishes and glasses in the kitchen and entertain in an informal manner, I found it was wasted space as a dining room. By considering usage I actually gained extra space for my all-important main guidance center and study.

The living room is generally where gatherings occur, either for socializing, flopping down at the end of a day, or playing. You may have the advantage of a separate family room in your home.

There are hints to decrease the energy you need to expend keeping things clean.

Placing furniture on casters lets you easily move them around for cleaning and rearranging. I have been dubbed the master of rearrangement and casters have allowed me to earn this title!

My son has a weekly chore of dusting my collection of pottery that is on the fireplace mantle. He gets his allowance and I get to keep my pottery out on display without expending energy for upkeep.

Two color-coordinated, plastic crates contain family games and toys which I rotate weekly. These are on casters too, and make end-of-day cleaning a breeze.

Eons ago I banished the proverbial coffee table from my living room. No one seemed to miss it except to complain they had no place to put their dishes. When I heard that was the main complaint, I knew I was on the right track. One less piece of furniture to polish and dust and no "forgotten dishes" in the living room.

Bedrooms are traditionally located on an upper floor in two-story homes, but this may not be the best location if mobility and decreased energy are issues. If you have the advantage of a den and living room on the main floor, consider turning the den into your bedroom. By using the guest or entrance closet for your clothes and adding a coat tree for guests, you can overcome the problem of not having a closet. A day-bed with proper mattress can look fine if space is an issue.

A widow found that by purchasing a standing wardrobe and day-bed for her den, she had a closet and still had room for her two comfy chairs. The room maintained the essence of an informal den while doubling as her bedroom.

A family acquaintance did not have a den to turn into a bedroom, so his solution was to have a sleeping sofa in the living room with two chifforobes for his clothes. They looked like antiques and blended with the end table that doubled as his bedside stand. A neighbor would come in nightly to open the sofa-bed and in the morning to close it. Amazing: by day a living room and by night a bedroom.

By keeping the furniture in the bedroom simple, you will simplify your cleaning. Casters for the bed are a must, as well as comforters in lieu of bedspreads. Comforters act both as spread and cover and are a snap to make tidy.

A headboard is beautiful. However, you may want to consider eliminating it and filling the wall space with wall-hangings or pictures. Remember, surfaces require up-keep, so think twice about whether you really need that headboard.

A beautiful heirloom tablecloth was sitting in the linen closet for years. During a spring cleaning session, my neighbor came across it while helping me with my chores. She made a passing comment that it was a shame such a wonderful work of art was hidden away. Two weeks later I purchased two wooden dowels and had my neighbor stitch the top and bottom of the tablecloth to the dowels. In place of my headboard I now have my heirloom tablecloth hanging.

In a child's bedroom, a wall of cork or series of cork boards eliminates damage to wall surfaces. Posters and memorabilia are tacked on the cork instead, meaning touch-ups or repainting do not have to be done as often.

Built-in bookcases, bureaus, desks and beds help keep

furniture in perimeter placement. There are even designs which suspend everything off the floor for almost maintenance-free care. If built-ins are not possible, or to your liking, the mere choice of simplicity and perimeter furniture placement will be a plus.

A standard bed can be placed on foot blocks and will achieve the same effect of raising it to an energy-efficient level, with minimum cost and effort.

The closer the bath is to the bedrooms, the better. However, because they have a defined use and rarely can be moved or added without great expense, we are left pretty much at the mercy of the architect. Many older homes locate a single bath on the second (upper) story, which is quite convenient for the bedrooms, but a definite hurdle for the person with low energy or physical impairment. Running up the stairs every time you must use the facility causes fatigue. A lavatory on the main floor can greatly reduce the expenditure of energy.

Instead of receiving multiple, little gifts for the holiday season, a woman researched and asked for an electric stair-glide chair. Her family and friends were more than happy to give her what they called "the gift of energy." Installation coincided with a holiday, pot-luck appetizer party. There were smiles of joy all around and the children kept occupied with the new "toy."

FIXTURES AND MATERIALS SHOULD BE EASY TO CLEAN

Making any room work for you, instead of against you, can be quite a task. Take a look at the fixtures, materials, windows and floors in order to evaluate the level of energy you will need to maintain them.

Fixtures and materials that are easy to clean with a wipe of a sponge are best. Chrome is great and can sparkle with little care. Combination fiberglass tubs and showers come in one unit and eliminate the headaches of tile and grout. As pretty as shower or tub doors are, cleaning one is atrocious and time consuming. Opt for vinyl shower and tub curtains that can be replaced as soon as they become "scummy." They cost only a few dollars and come in a plentiful array of colors and patterns.

A neat trick I read about in a hints' column was that vinyl shower curtains can be washed in a washing machine with a large bath towel. Some vinegar added to the water helps remove the soap scum.

Porcelain sinks and toilet tops and formica or corian counters do not need scrubbing and keep their lustre. Stainless steel in the kitchen is easy maintenance and will not chip.

Once again, vinyl is great floor covering for kitchen, baths and entrances. The ever-shine varieties are just that — forever shining. You can choose from a range of costs and quality.

Window treatments can be found to suit any taste and budget. The less there is hanging, the easier the cleaning. You can have privacy without shades and drapes. Designer mini-blinds, with or without matching valances, can solve this problem in either fabric or vinyl. Vertical blinds are another option, although tend to be more costly. Both the mini-blinds and verticals can blend with any decor, so your personal taste does not have to be compromised.

If you have frosted windows in the bath, you do not need curtains, blinds, or shades for privacy. Most mail-order catalogs and hardware stores carry do-it-yourself "frosting" for window panes.

By hanging two plastic-coated wire shelves over my toilet, I am able to store towels and miscellaneous items such as toilet paper, shampoo, powder and tissue within easy reach. This clears my under-sink cabinet for cleaning supplies and personals. The cleaning supplies are kept in a plastic carry-all, just right for toting to any other room in the house.

"Sponge-up" as you go along by keeping a large sponge on the sink. It is surprising how you can avoid heavy scrubbing by wiping with a swipe every time you use the room.

Every time I shower, I use a scrub pad that I keep in the hanging shower caddy to wipe accumulated soap scum. Do a little every day and you will not have to do any heavy scouring. Everyone in the house follows this same routine.

Keep a toilet brush by the bowl and swish frequently. Accumulation of stains and mess here can mean tiring cleaning — on your knees. Try an in-tank, every flush cleaner that is environmentally safe.

ADEQUATE LIGHTING AND FIXTURE PLACEMENT IS IMPORTANT

It is very important to know that inadequate lighting and improper placement is both bad for the eyes and stress-inducing. Optimum illumination and placement of light fixtures creates working ease and decreases tension. Ceiling lighting is best because it saves on cleaning and comes in a variety of styles and with variable cost. There is even a greater choice of types of illumination, such as incandescent versus florescent. Put in ceiling fixtures anywhere you can. Wiring is generally inexpensive and easy to do, even by you or family and friends. There are many how-to books on the market.

A combination paddle fan and light will do double-duty. The many styles fit into almost any decor and price range. Cathedral ceilings are not the only place for them. Movement of air and good lighting can be used anywhere.

Recessed lights and track lighting offer the best bet for little or no maintenance. Unfortunately, they are not always aesthetically pleasing and may be difficult to install if you are not buying/renting new construction.

CREATE LAUNDRY WORK SPACE
THAT IS ENERGY EFFICIENT

Tantamount to the frequency and number of loads of laundry you do is the work space necessary for this chore. You must create space in which to sort, fold and carry clothes.

Start with a rolling laundry cart, which can be purchased inexpensively at local department stores or through catalogs. You can easily roll to-and-from the laundry basket.

Make sure there is a flat surface for folding by the washer and dryer and somewhere to hang things. You can expend lots of energy traveling between places to fold or hang things.

Folding snack trays can be wheeled to the laundry area, opened and lined up to create a flat surface.

A friend's laundry facility was in the basement, so he laid a large piece of painted plywood across two folding chairs for his work space.

A piece of rope strung between two opposing surfaces can act as a mini-clothes line for drying or for hanger items.

Portable shirt stands made of light-weight aluminum can be found in most stores and in catalogs. They have adjustable arms that raise for hanging and drop for storage.

Hooks are multipurpose and great for various hanging needs.

Creating a comfortable and less stressful environment for the laundry is easier than you may think. Remembering the tenet to never stand when you can sit, a comfortable chair should be located in the laundry area. Instead of running to-and-fro between loads, sit and relax by reading, enjoying the radio or doing your favorite handcraft. All of a sudden laundry time can become a pleasant part of your day.

LANDSCAPE FOR LOW MAINTENANCE

Just as it is necessary to think and redirect your energies for the inside of your home, so must you take the time to survey the land around you. Outside work can be the most laborious and energy-threatening.

Your choices from the vast array of shrubbery, flowers and ground cover can directly effect how much energy you expend in care and upkeep. This does not mean things have to look stark and sparse, merely well-planned. Much of the surveying and planning can be done at home through the use of books and a little imagination. The local library will have many books to choose from and most nurseries are willing to take the time to discuss such issues. They also have many free merchandise pamphlets. Nurseries will, of course, be very glad to come out and do the surveying and planning for you, but usually the price is high.

Do not be daunted. On a nice day, take a slow stroll around your yard and take a good look at what is already there. A simple diagram is all that is needed to show approximate locations and names of the various plants and shrubs. You are not creating a work of art, so sketch away! Decide what you want to eliminate and where you want to add something. By doing this you can change your mind a thousand times merely by adding or subtracting from your diagram.

My ignorance about flora was astounding prior to owning my own home. The first place I started was my son's bookshelf, where I found a book on trees and greenery that I had purchased for elementary school use. It was perfect. We created a weekend project that not only provided me with my plot diagram, but refined my son's reference skills. A picnic lunch topped off a fun and productive day.

When you pick out shrubbery, choose double-duty varieties. If the shrubs will be fairly low and spreading, they can act as ground cover and do not need trimming. You can even bring in color, for many shrubs come in red hues.

Hedging shrubs need some degree of maintenance for

annual shaping, while others require very little. There are bushes which grow fairly wild, tall and spreading. Forsythia comes to mind and it provides screening, privacy and a beautiful yellow color in early spring.

Trees provide shade and can be quite majestic. Each state has a Department of Environmental Management as well as a Division of Fisheries and Game for assistance in locating free trees; but be prepared — they will be fledglings, not full grown. Trees can also solve drainage problems, such as weeping willows for areas where water pools. Once again, pruning is necessary, but not prohibitive.

Grass is great, but requires mowing, reseeding and fertilizing for best results. If you have any embankments or steep hills, think about utilizing ground cover shrubbery, bark mulch, or wildflower and clover seeding instead of grass. Both options simply require that nature take its course, not your spent energies.

My family invested in a beautifully designed patio area using patio blocks. The area of grass was significantly cut down by doing this and there were no more hassles with unsteady chairs and picnic tables due to the uneven ground.

Flowers are beautiful and do require care and attention. The best bet is to have annuals planted if you want flower beds along with your shrubs. However, the best of both worlds can be had by using large or hanging flower pots and boxes. You can change the colors and varieties seasonally with low maintenance. This saves the knees and back. Initial cost may be a bit more due to the purchase of pots and soil along with the plants, but the long term benefits are worth it.

When purchasing any type of gardening or nursery products, always ask for help to load your items and have someone waiting at home to unload. Most items are not only bulky, but incredibly heavy.

The purchase of a large, plastic trash can with lid can assist in long-term storage of soil and you can control the amount for transfer easily.

A sturdy child's red wagon is great for transporting your tools, soil and potting items.

When watering hanging plants, remove the plant from the hanger and water at a level where you do not have to reach up with your filled watering can.

A hose with a sprinkler attachment means you can water your planting beds by simply turning on your outdoor faucet. A spray nozzle will accomplish a similar task.

A neighborhood child might love to earn a few dollars during the spring and summer doing yard-work. Call your local school principal and guidance counselor for names if there are no children in your immediate neighborhood.

The outdoors can be a quiet and beautiful haven in which to sit and enjoy all that nature has to offer. You will be surprised at how rejuvenated you can feel with just a few minutes spent outside the confines of your home. When mood and spirit are improved, your energies will be enhanced, especially if your outdoor escape is virtually worry-free and easy to care for.

BE PURCHASE OR RENTAL SMART

When in the market for a new place, be open and honest about your limitations. The options available are numerous; from that romantic, gothic mansion to a studio walk-up. Eventually dollar availability becomes the key to what is affordable and you will quickly realize that persistence and resourcefulness pay off.

Energy conservation and limitations are relevant issues when looking for something new. Choose not only what appeals, but what is practical. Be picky. Picky means you will ultimately enjoy being at home because you have chosen wisely.

Single family homes can be large or small and run the spectrum in cost. Choose a home that locates much of your daily living on the main floor. If the laundry is in the basement, can it be moved upstairs to a closet or into the bathroom? Can a chair glide be used on an existing staircase if the only bath is on an upper level?

A ranch-style presents many stellar qualities because everything is accessible on one floor.. Cape Cods offer a bedroom on the first floor and you have the option of not using the second story until the extra bedrooms and bath become necessary.

Look at the entrances of a home to determine if easily accessed. If you are in the snow belt, is there a long driveway that will need shoveling? Can you get into your kitchen or storage area with groceries without having to climb lots of stairs? Do you have to carry heavy loads a great distance from the car? Many main entrances are designed with decorative steps, which are appealing to the eye but definitely drain energy. Steps need maintenance and upkeep and can be quite dangerous when slippery.

A garage that is attached to the house is wonderful because it offers protection from the elements. You can directly enter the the house from inside. If the garage offers access through the basement, be sure to check out how many stairs you will have to climb and if it can accommodate a chair glide.

My attached garage gives me access through the basement but requires a climb to the main floor. The stairs are straight, not curved, and a chair glide can be installed when it becomes necessary. In the interim, I have rigged a pulley system from the bottom of the stairs to the top. This allows me to load parcels into a carrying basket, flip an electrical switch and off the packages go. If the electricity goes out I can manually operate it much like a clothesline.

SERIOUSLY CONSIDER HOUSING ALTERNATIVES

Alternatives to single family homes can be financially more appealing and energy-saving. If your budget will not allow for a purchase, then renting or living with family are other options.

During your search for an appropriate rental unit, use the same guidelines as for any home you would live in. There are additional considerations to be aware of when you rent an apartment.

Reliable elevators in apartment buildings are imperative. Talk to some of the neighbors and ask about it.

Trash chutes located on each floor can save carrying loads to the dumpster or refuse cans.

If there is a laundry facility in the building, where is it and when are the peak times for usage. Reliability of the machines will save trips to the laundromat. Some apartment buildings have laundry chutes, so check it out.

On-site parking will make life much easier. If it's off-site parking, you must know how far away your spot is and the terrain to be traveled to reach it. On-site garage parking is optimum. The energy expended is minimal and there are no hassles with cleaning off snow and ice. Also, in hot or arid climates, your car will remain cool.

Condominiums are numerous and offer varying services for fee. There are condominiums which also allow rentals. When considering condominium living, make sure that you find out about your rights, privileges and fees. Many condominium associations do not extend various services and facility usage to rentals.

Special amenities for fee, such as pool and other recreational facilities, will mean a higher maintenance fee per month. Assess whether you will actually use these facilities or be paying for what you will never use. It may be worth having all the special recreational possibilities on site if you have children. It could mean not paying extra membership fees for their extracurricular activities and you do not have to transport!

When I relocated from my large, single family home, I decided that condominium living would be the answer. It took me the better part of a year to locate one which met my energy and physical needs, without paying unnecessary costs. The association fee was for outside maintenance and landscaping only and has only moderately increased per year. I certainly could not justify paying for recreational facilities I would never use. The insurance alone to maintain these would also guarantee a hefty dollar increase in fees annually.

Retirement communities present a unique opportunity

for relocation. Many of the newer communities are now open to individuals with physical and medical restrictions. "Younger olders" are also opting for the more carefree living of these communities. There is the added appeal of the availability of mixed rentals, ownership and styles to suit many tastes and budgets. A plus is that services ranging from laundering, on-site health care and transportation can be contracted.

Nursing homes can be a viable option if your physical capabilities are quite compromised and your health status tenuous. Retirement homes are changing to meet the demands of the consumer and do not have to resemble the sterile, impersonal nursing homes of years past. Once again, be picky. If this type of housing is necessary, make sure you evaluate how the home meets your daily living standards and desires.

Look for cleanliness in both the structural upkeep and the residents.

Make sure the rooms are readily accessible to nursing stations and recreation areas, with no "forgotten rooms."

A cheery, lively and inviting atmosphere generally means both staff and residents are content and happy.

Evaluate the design and layout of the rooms to see if they will accommodate your particular living style. Many places will allow you to either totally or partially furnish the room yourself.

Check out the services available to residents, including transportation, trips and on-site activities. Programs with local school children are wonderful and provide both parties with the chance to interact and learn. Many of these programs involve tutoring, senior pen-pals, social visits and walk-mates.

Recreational and exercise programs are important and take into consideration varying levels of energy and abilities. Make sure they are an integral part of daily life.

Look for sunrooms, porches and grounds in order to bring some of the good old outdoors into your life.

LIVING WITH OTHERS CAN LEAD TO GREATER INDEPENDENCE

In today's social and economic climate, more and more people are finding it necessary to cohabit. For the person with low energy reserves, this can be a boon.

Living with others can mean family, roommates or a planned community. By sharing the load of daily tasks your energy-sapping activities will be lessened, or even eliminated. In turn, you can take up the chores best suited to your abilities and endurance levels. Of course there will be episodes of friction and this cannot be avoided; however, the positives generally outweigh the problems.

After nine years of marriage our family friend found herself divorced and on her own to raise her family. All of a sudden the days became unmanageable, with overwhelming psychological and physical demands. Her deficient energy reserves were taxed to their limit and illness was around the corner. The solution came one day when an acquaintance found he was on unemployment and needed a place to stay until he was working again. The opportunity presented itself, so she offered her spare room in return for various household and chauffeur duties. It worked so well, he has remained on as helper, boarder and friend, even though he is working!

Cooperation and shared living are invaluable resources for anyone with decreased energy and limitations. Privacy is gained due to the increased independence that comes from productively pacing yourself.

BE NEIGHBORHOOD SMART
WHEN CHOOSING HOUSING

Almost as important as your home itself is accessibility to necessary services and neighborhood. You can be as energy efficient and paced as you want at home, but valuable ground will be lost if you live great distances from support services and businesses. A well-designed house or routine may mean you never carry groceries up stairs; but if the market is thirty minutes away you defeat the purpose.

If possible, choose a housing location that has the greatest access to those places you frequent often. These include markets, retail stores, gasoline, post office, bank, barber or hairdresser, cleaners, laundromat and restaurant. You can check out many other services as well.

If mass transportation is near, you will not be isolated. A simple phone call to the local mass transit authority will give you time tables and information. Using a bus or train for an errand can double as an outing for children, elders and friends.

Many local senior centers provide mini-bus transportation to medical appointments, markets and shopping plazas. This is also true of local agencies for the handicapped. Do not let the name of the organization stop you from utilizing services that can be valuable time and energy savers.

Home delivery of groceries is provided by some smaller markets and worth the extra cost. Also, in some parts of the country, markets are instituting phone-in shopping. You are provided with a home-list of items with the choice of pick-up or delivery. The number of supermarkets with drive-up windows for small orders are also increasing.

Many markets are now providing sit-down motorized, shopping scooters. Use them.

If there is a market with varied businesses under the same roof — or in the same plaza — shopping can be coupled with other errands.

Check with your local post office about purchasing stamps from your mail carrier. If your box is located away from the house, ask about door-to-door delivery.

Local businesses such as plumbing, heating and electrical can make life a lot easier.

The proximity of neighbors is important, especially on those "bad days." Mutual concern and shared respect with neighbors comes with time, but is a valuable seed to be sowed. Informal neighborhood networks are commonly set up for things such as marketing, banking and postal runs. Availing yourself of these networks, and sharing in them will greatly reduce your energy expenditure.

A young mother, compromised by pulmonary problems, found that one of her neighbors made a weekly run to the produce stand. While talking together one day, she asked her neighbor if she would be willing to pick up items for her when she went. Now, at the beginning of each week, her neighbor stops by for the list and money. A trip is saved.

When I am going on an errand I phone my neighbor to see if she wants anything. Since I've started this, I find that I too get a call when she is going on an errand. Our mutual consideration helps both of us but we do not feel obliged to call. We know that when we can, we will.

One morning there was a knock on my door. My recently widowed neighbor from the condominium unit in back came by to check on me. She and I have a standing joke that we are the only ones up with the birds. We both start our day at dawn and turn on our kitchen lights. Living in the condominium complex we can see the other's light. She knew of my illness and on this particular day she became concerned because she did not see my light. Indeed, I had not felt well and was dreading the drive to the doctor's office. She insisted on driving me and later in the day brought over some delicious Italian cookies.

LEARN TO BE ARCHITECTURE WISE

Not only does the person with low energy have to be concerned about home, but also about coping with architecture elsewhere. By learning to be architecture wise you can anticipate obstacles that may present themselves. Anticipation leads to prevention and increases the chances for energy conservation. When possible, choose those places best suited to your needs.

Call ahead if you are unfamiliar with a particular building you may be going to. Ask about parking, steps, elevators, seating arrangements and bathroom facilities.

If a wait is anticipated, make sure you will have a place to sit. Many discount stores and catalogs sell lightweight, folding stools. I carry one with me for those unexpected stops.

If you know there will be a particular problem with a certain location, but it is unavoidable to go there, make some pre-arrangements. Most owners and employees, with advance notice, are more than willing to accommodate.

EDUCATE OTHERS ABOUT YOUR NEEDS

Most times people are pleased and flattered to know you trust them enough to share the information about your special needs. Another person cannot read your mind or know your particular situation unless told about it. Informed decision making can take place if all the cards are on the table.

Sometimes you will not want to reveal personal information to someone. If you cannot effect a change in plans you know will be an architectural and geographic problem for you, it is best to decline.

I had repeatedly accompanied an acquaintance on what was supposed to be a quick errand only to find we made, on-the-average, five different stops. Most required climbing stairs and offered no place to sit and rest. At first I did not want to let her know that these stops were exhausting for me. She was so nice to be with. I began declining her invitations and found out from a mutual friend she was quite hurt. All turned out well when I made a point to explain my condition and limits. She was appalled to think she could have made me ill because she ran me ragged. I had done her a great disservice without realizing it and caused myself harm in the interim.

When running errands or going out with someone, have them drop you off at an entrance so you will not have to do extra walking. It is amazing how those "little" stops can tire you out after they accumulate over an entire day.

In essence, ease in living can be enhanced, despite those daily annoyances and frustrations. By incorporating energy conserving, architectural ideas and design into your home and living, you can more easily pace yourself. And if you are architecture wise, excursions will be truly enjoyable.

Just A Hop, Skip And A Jump Away — 5

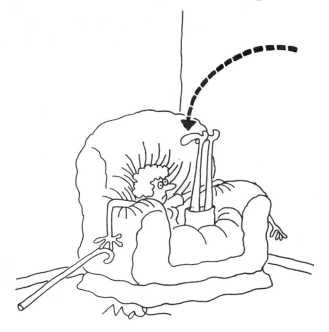

GOOD POSTURE SAVES ENERGY

EFFECTIVE BODY MECHANICS MAKE MOVING THINGS EASIER AND SAFER

FLEXIBILITY IS A KEY TO ENERGY CONSERVATION

USING THE TELEPHONE SAVES YOUR ENERGY

MANEUVERING

Depleted energy levels need not leave you home-bound. It is good for the spirit to spend time outdoors, to experience a change of scenery, to visit friends and travel to new places. It may indeed be possible to get someplace with enough remaining energy to do something. Planning will ensure that you spend your energy efficiently and a commitment to periodic rests will give your body time to recharge. In addition there are techniques of personal movement that help conserve energy. Anticipating your needs and the transportation services available will make travel easier and more pleasant.

GOOD POSTURE SAVES ENERGY

When your body parts are properly aligned, your muscles are able to relax. Proper posture balances the weight of your head and limbs on the skeletal frame; gravity assists in keeping the alignment. Postures that put body parts out of alignment cause muscles to tense and work against gravity to maintain an unnatural position. The head and back should be straight and the arms relaxed at the shoulders. This is important whether you are at rest or active.

The design of a chair affects your sitting posture. To facilitate correct posture, a chair should have full seat support, armrests, and back support. It is important that your feet rest on the floor. Sitting in such a chair will align your body parts and allow your muscles to relax.

To rise more easily from sitting, make this technique a habit: scoot forward to the edge of the seat, place your feet about 12 inches apart for stability, lean forward, bending at the hips, and look up as you stand up.

It is difficult to sit down or raise yourself from a seat that is too low. Someone of average height will find that a seat height of 22 to 24 inches is far easier to manage than one of 18 inches or less. More generally a seat that comes only to your knee when you stand beside it will be more of a struggle than one a few inches higher. While higher seats are easier to get into and out of, the extra height means your feet will not reach the floor when you sit. So consider raising toilet seats, your bed, the telephone chair — seats you often get on and off. The chairs where you work and rest should provide support for your feet so if raised for accessibility, use a box or footstool for good posture.

Soft living room sofas can be especially difficult to get up from and may encourage a slouch rather than proper posture. A board under the seat cushions will make the seat firmer and pillows may improve the back support; however, sitting in such furniture is probably best avoided altogether.

Furniture can be raised on wooden blocks. Chair leg extenders and raised toilet seats can be mail ordered. Be sure that the furniture you raise is stable.

By raising your bed you will not only make it easier — literally — to get up in the morning, you will find it easier to change the sheets.

When you work at a task, the position of your materials can cause you to use bad posture or assist you in maintaining good posture. Analyze your work positions. Are you bending over? If so, you need to raise the work surface. Do you work with your shoulders hunched?

Lower the work height. Do you hold your head inclined forward? The problem may be with your chair back or your work may be too low. The correct position for your work allows you to keep your neck and back straight.

Prop your book on a pillow or book rack to avoid bending over when you read.

Adjust the car seat, as good posture will mean more relaxed driving.

A computer keyboard can be lowered to a more comfortable typing height with a sliding tray mounted under the desk.

EFFECTIVE BODY MECHANICS
MAKE MOVING THINGS EASIER AND SAFER

Using good body mechanics is important when you have to move or lift objects. The large joints, those closest to the trunk, are the strongest and the most stable and should be used whenever possible. To pick up large objects, bend at the knees and hips. Smaller objects should be picked up with both hands, palms up. This distributes the weight between both hands and wrists and to the stronger elbow joint. Slide rather than lift. Push heavy objects with the weight of your body, using your hip or shoulder. Better yet — put everything on wheels!

Carry a pocketbook over your forearm rather than in your hand. This shifts the weight from your wrist and hand joints to the elbow and shoulder.

Use tote bags with long straps to carry over your shoulder.

You can spare your back by using your feet. Kick bottom drawers and cabinets closed. Mop up spills by dropping a paper towel and wiping with your toe.

Good posture saves energy when you stand and walk; therefore, proper fitting is very important for canes, walkers, and crutches. Seek professional advice when choosing an ambulation aid and learn the techniques for safe use.

When you walk, set a moderate pace. Rushing uses excessive energy and, surprisingly, so does an exceptionally slow pace.

Overweight individuals are using extra energy to move the burden of extra pounds. Keeping your body weight down is basic to the conservation of energy.

Cargo carrying while using an ambulation aid requires some kind of satchel. Cane users will want a shoulder bag or wheeled bag. There are small pocketbooks designed to strap onto T-handled canes. Crutch pouches can be filled with a few items, such as eyeglasses and a billfold, but should not be overloaded.

Two bags will improve your balance; however a knapsack is preferable for heavy items. Carrier bags for walkers will handle several light items. These various bags can be made at home or purchased.

Remember that carrying extra weight in any manner will decrease your endurance.

An ambulation aid should always be kept within reach. You may want a cane clip to clamp your cane to a table, desk, or wall. A wheelchair user who ambulates sometimes should have a cane or crutch holder on the chair.

Powered scooters help conserve energy. They run on electric batteries which are recharged overnight. More compact than wheelchairs they can be used in many settings. Good trunk control and balance are necessary to use a scooter safely. Ask your physician or therapist for guidance before purchasing one.

There are sling seats designed to fasten to a walker, converting the ambulation aid to a chair and thereby allowing you to sit down anywhere. For those who do not use an aid for walking but like the idea of a take-along chair, there are cane seats. These are made of lightweight aluminum, fold compactly, and are handy for the bus stop.

Your outings should include scheduled rests. The extra exertion of your activities may require more frequent rests than usual. It is important to recognize your body's signs of fatigue and respond to them. Make time to sit down and relax.

The weather influences the energy you spend maneuvering. When the temperature is either very hot or cold, the body directs energy to warming or cooling itself, leaving less available for activity. The heart works harder meeting the body's increased oxygen demand. Air quality affects the heart's function, too. When air pollution is bad or when it is hot or cold, you must reduce your activity level. As important as it is to plan ahead, there has to be flexibility in your planning to allow for unexpected changes in the weather.

FLEXIBILITY IS A KEY TO ENERGY CONSERVATION

When the weather is hot you need to keep in cool places as much as possible. Dress in light clothing and drink a lot of fluids to aid your body in keeping its chemical balance and conserving energy.

In cold weather, wear layers of clothing and include a hat and scarf because much body heat is lost from the head and neck region. A muffler around your neck and chin also serves to warm the air you breathe.

Ice and snow call for a good measure of common sense. Do not risk injury by going out when you shouldn't. Delegate your responsibilities. When you do go outdoors wear boots with non-skid treads. There are special tips made for canes and crutches for security in the snow or on ice. Some have deep treads and go on over the standard tips; others have steel prongs which can be flipped up when the weather improves.

Driving can be a pleasant, energy-efficient activity — when your seat is comfortable, the weather is fair, traffic is light, and you are taking a familiar route. Conversely, driving can be very stressful if you are late, lost, or stuck in traffic. Such tension is exhausting. Apply the energy conservation principles of delegation, planning, flexibility, and proper positioning to driving. Further consider these specific suggestions:

Allow extra time.

Get good directions and look at a map before you leave.

Avoid rush hour.

Have your car serviced regularly.

Have duplicate keys made.

Adapt the seat for good posture.

Keep sunglasses in the car.

Following a stroke or other changes in physical status, it may be necessary to be retrained in driving. Sometimes one needs to learn to drive with adapted controls such as hand operated brakes. There is a small but growing group of therapists specializing in driver education for the disabled. A state government office or a hospital specializing in rehabilitation could help you find a driving instructor.

If your low energy level is a chronic condition, you may be eligible for a handicapped license plate or placard. By telephoning the state registry of motor vehicles, you can obtain an application. Your physician will need to complete part of the application, attesting to the degree and permanence of your disability. In the case of an "invisible handicap" it is particularly important that the physician document the extent of your impairment. The advantage of having a handicapped plate or placard, of course, is access to reserved parking places near entrances to stores, restaurants, and other public buildings.

USING THE TELEPHONE SAVES YOUR ENERGY

It is important to educate yourself about the services available in your area. Transportation services for the elderly, chronically ill, and disabled are improving all the time. Many areas now have senior vans and wheelchair buses. Use the telephone and telephone book to investigate what your community offers. Compare the services. Do some have no-smoking policies? Do some have better heating and air conditioning? Does the local taxi company give senior discounts? Your health insurance may cover transportation costs.

If you live in a rural area where such services are not established, a little creativity may be necessary to handle your transportation needs. Through the church, the "Y," or the school, you could find a responsible teenager to be your driver. You might barter with a neighbor to exchange services. You could provide dinner in exchange for running errands.

Sometimes all you have to do is ask.

We know a woman in Virginia who hired her neighbor's grandson to take her shopping. He drove her car.

Four sisters who live in a small town in rural Ohio routinely call each other before going shopping to see who needs what. It's a long drive to the store so when one sister goes, she shops for the others too.

Vacation planning begins with telephoning. Find out in advance about available services and emergency medical aid for each leg of your trip. Careful planning from home can prevent your being stranded in a hotel without an elevator, a bus without air conditioning or a bathroom on the second floor.

One rich source of free information is the public library. Medium and large libraries have reference librarians whose sole job it is to help you find the answers to your questions. They will deal with you over the telephone, saving you a trip to the library. Reference libraries have a great deal of information about travel and these resources are just a telephone call away.

If you will be traveling by air you should call ahead to the airport to arrange for a wheelchair and free baggage handling. Even if you do not use a wheelchair at home, it can save you a lot of walking in an airport. There is no reason to begin your trip fatigued from the walk to the gate.

If you are thinking of taking a tour, ask a lot of questions — about who carries the luggage, how often they take breaks, special diets, how early they leave each morning, and such. Look for established tour groups which specialize in elderly clients. There are disabled groups that plan vacations also.

Just as you can use a wheelchair to negotiate the airport, you may want a scooter to do sightseeing. Disney World is fairly buzzing with visitors who rent electric scooters to tour Epcot and the Magic Kingdom.

Another way to plan a vacation is to go with someone who is physically able. Such joint vacations give you a chance to travel with the reassurance that you will have help when you need it.

It had been years since I returned to Newport, R.I., my old college campus and haunts. My son and I decided it would be the perfect get-away on a forthcoming Saturday. For him, getting into the car and making sure he brought his spending money were the only prerequisites. For me, a lot more thought and planning would be necessary to assure a good day for all.

I phoned the main office of the college. I needed to know current information on the location of visitor and handicapped parking, the layout of buildings and the availability of places to rest on campus. They were so helpful and arranged for a special parking permit to be picked up at the switchboard. There was handicapped parking, but not all buildings had lots. This permit would allow us to park at the front entrances of these buildings. They forwarded a campus map, complete with "rest and relax" markings and accessible bathrooms. Two of the buildings did not have elevators, so they arranged to have a tour guide for my son, while I waited on the main level.

Knowing that we would also like to sight-see, I contacted the state Department of Travel and Tourism (an 800 number). There were many new attractions. Each brochure came with a number to call for more information and I contacted those we were interested in. They readily gave parking, elevator and restroom information. Restaurants were more than helpful regarding parking, accessible restrooms, special seating (type or space) and food restrictions. They indicated that as long as they knew ahead of time, there would be no problem. Asking to speak to the manager or proprietor was the key.

Newport is an island and my son loves to walk along the shore. Since there is no way for me to gauge my energy reserves, I asked a friend to come along. Should I get tired, there would be someone to take over while I sat and rested. My day would be enjoyable because I would not get exhausted, my son could be as exuberant as he wanted and we had the added bonus of sharing our day with a friend. Sharing the driving was nice as well.

Prior to leaving, I ran down my check list of "necessities", which I carry any time I leave the house for more than half a day. There is a backpack with a full change of clothes, a thermos with cold water, a zip-lock bag with dried fruit or cereal, and my medical dressing supplies (kept in a special cosmetics pouch). In the trunk of my car I always have an old pair of sneakers, a blanket, washcloth, paper towels and emergency car supplies. By getting my gas tank filled the day before, having my oil checked and tire pressure tested, there are no last minute hassles to sap my energy.

A good time was had by all and the next day-trip was already being planned.

When you pack for travel, go light on the clothes and

generous on the medical supplies. Take a few comfortable outfits and shoes. Be sure you have all the medicines you might need. Use the telephone to locate the nearest pharmacy and to contact the local home health care agency if appropriate.

Wear a medic alert bracelet. You can also take along a medical summary in your purse or wallet. These precautions can help insure that you get appropriate medical treatment in an emergency.

I can remember the first time I took a vacation on an airplane. After the excitement of making the flight reservations, the reality of what I was undertaking took hold. First, I would be away from my established center of medical care, my physician and my home medical supplier. What if I needed a doctor while I was out of state; or worse what if I needed hospitalization? My medical dressing supplies alone would take up half an airplane! What if I ran out? Prescriptions were another problem. How would I be able to get my luggage from place to place without exhausting myself before I even took off? Transportation was no problem at home, between friends, my car and handicapped placard; but what about there? Was traveling alone the way to go?

Never to be daunted, I decided that if my life could be paced and managed at home, I certainly could manage to plan a vacation. The key would have to be pre-planning and lots of phone calls.

I decided that one whole week would have to be given over to accomplishing this task. Since medical concerns were the most imperative and had the potential to cause the most problems, I started there. A phone call to my physician proved a bit more time consuming than I thought. Three calls and two days later (I was not ill and it was not an emergency) I was able to talk to my doctor. I told him my plans and asked if he would please write a short letter outlining my condition and treatment regimens; give me prescriptions to get filled for the time I would be away; and to provide me with a name of a contact physician in the area I would be visiting. He agreed and stated he was glad I was giving him enough time to do this. Within the week I had everything I requested.

Once I had the away-physician's name, I phoned him to explain how and why I was referred to him. It took two calls and persistence to get past the secretary. She did not want to let me speak to the doctor myself, insisting my own physician had to call. I firmly stated that my doctor had directed me to call and that if after talking to me he wanted to follow-up by contacting my physician, then fine. It was definitely a good thing to do, for it turned out that during the time I would be in his area, he was going to be on vacation himself! He gave me the name of his partner and told me he would give him my information. To be of further assistance, he provided me with the name of the senior resident at the hospital, who would be in on my case as well, should I need hospitalization. Never the trusting sort, I sent off a letter to them with a copy of my doctor's summary and a reminder of our conversation. Of course I would carry with me an outline of my medical history, pertinent laboratory information, my doctor's summary and referral physician's names and numbers.

Next I contacted my home medical supplier, explained my vacation plans and asked the best way to handle my dressing supplies. It turned out they could direct-mail them to the address of my destination. They also gave me the name of an area home medical supplier who could assist in an emergency. A written letter was forwarded to me showing my patient status and the physician orders. If I preferred, they would deliver the supplies to my home and I could take them with me. It was suggested that I carry two days worth anyway, "just in case." I opted for the mailing, breathing a sigh of relief for much less baggage.

A call to the airport public relations supervisor provided me with lots of information. There were porters available to transport my luggage to whatever airline desk was necessary. All I had to do was be at the main terminal entrance. Wheelchairs were also provided. It was suggested that I let the senior flight attendant know so I could avoid the tiring wait at the gate for embarking. They could seat me earlier. Also the airline would notify the airport at my destination and have a porter and wheelchair waiting at the gate. Easy!

The Department of Travel and Tourism was more than happy to send me information on places of interest and maps. This required an 800 phone call. By phoning the state's Department of Transportation, I was able to obtain information on the various forms of transportation available, timetables and commuter maps. The Department of Motor Vehicles stated that my placard was not usable in their state, but that a special, temporary placard could be obtained if I sent a notarized copy of my state's approval. They were quick to point out that each state had different requirements. My local library was able to give me these various department numbers.

Knowing that I would be meeting friends at the other end, I decided that traveling alone was fine, especially with all the prior preparations made. By asking a neighbor to drive me to the airport and to pick me up on my return, all was set.

I had a marvelous time, did not have to call the referred physician and even did some of my own sightseeing, using the transportation information I had obtained prior to leaving. I felt as independent and self-reliant as I do at home, pacing myself without the added worries of uncertainty. Pre-planning and zillions of phone calls were well worth the effort for a truly relaxing vacation.

Vacation should be a time of renewal, not a time of stress and fatigue. You may find that a day trip fulfills your need to get away without the hassles an overnight stay can entail. A day at a local park or museum may be refreshing and easy to manage.

Finally we remind you that you can enjoy the outdoors without leaving home. Sit in a chair outside and feel the warmth of the sun and the coolness of the breeze. Even indoors, turn a chair toward the window and watch the birds and the clouds. It is good for the soul to keep in touch with the natural world and low energy levels need not prevent it.

Practical Partying — 6

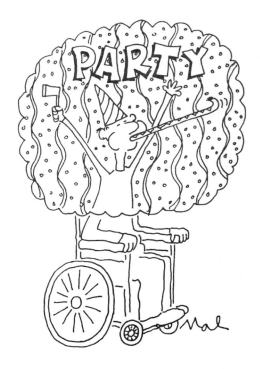

SPREAD SOCIALIZING THROUGHOUT THE WEEK

DO NOT ISOLATE YOURSELF

CANDID COMMUNICATION IS VITAL

**ALTERNATIVE METHODS
FOR SEXUAL ENJOYMENT**

LEISURE AND PLAY WILL REAP REWARDS

SOCIALIZING

You are finally able to sit and sift through today's mail. Your energy is gone, as you knew it would be from years of living with your condition. Hidden within the array of bills is an unfamiliar handwriting. It turns out to be an invitation to a business dinner next weekend. Of all days it would have to be when you are scheduled to do the marketing and have a doctor's appointment. Ending with a late night would more than sap your weeks' energy, not to mention the day's. How can you possibly attend?

Even though retired, you and your spouse keep quite active. Bridge and bowling get you out to meet friends. This Saturday the bowling league decided to have a postgame get-together at a fancy restaurant, one hour away from home. It promises to be quite a bash. However, the distance and back-to-back activities could prove quite hectic, especially when you know your energy levels are low. Do you choose just one event or attend both?

Being widowed and frail you find you spend most of your time sitting alone. You now live in an elderly housing complex instead of your house of forty-five years. Family is far away and friends are not as able to get around as they once did. The hours drag.

The intimate enjoyment that you and your spouse once shared seems to have vaporized with the progressiveness of your joint pain and fatigue. There is an emptiness you cannot bridge. Is this all there is from now on?

You keep saying that you need time to recover from your heart attack. This is only an excuse to avoid the time when you and your spouse will once again share a bed. You cannot possibly surmount the overwhelming fear of dying while making love and you are afraid of the memory of crushing pain. How can you ever enjoy this tender part of life again? How can you erase that anguished look on your spouse's face?

So many scars and now permanent tubes exist on what used to be a body you knew so well. Intimacy and revealing yourself to anyone seems impossible. Who wants damaged goods? Where has all that pride and self-worth gone ... and how do you regain it?

Perhaps some of the feelings expressed in these vignettes are familiar to you. When fatigue and low energy are hallmarks of your day-to-day life, it is easy to despair. But remember to make time for fun. Do not put fun on a shelf to collect dust! Leisure must be built into every day. Both the mind and body will benefit if fun becomes part of your routine. Events can be evaluated and reworked so that you can optimize your energy and fun.

EDUCATE ABOUT YOUR NEEDS AND LIMITATIONS

First and foremost, educate your friends and family about your needs and limitations. No one can read your mind even if you wish they could. The retired couple represented in our vignette is facing the dilemma of choice between activities with friends. If both events are attended, exhaustion for one spouse will be the result. If one event is chosen, misunderstanding and misinterpretation is possible. By taking the time to explain your restrictions, needs and concerns, this dilemma need not arise.

How to tell someone about your special needs may seem difficult. We have found that the more candid and direct you are, especially about a "hidden" disability, the better. Choose a relaxing and private place to converse — a place you are most comfortable. Do not hesitate to practice your "spiel" ahead of time. Say things out loud so that you not only think the words, but hear them as well. Be frank about what you want to talk about and why you want to share this information. It may be awkward at first, but your revelations may actually foster a positive closeness brought about by honesty. Suddenly the times in the past you opted "out" of activities or left early are understandable.

There was a time when I elected to tell a new acquaintance from work about my "no" to a skiing weekend. We were sitting in my den with a fire going. It was good that I was wearing a turtle-neck jersey, because I had hives and blotches. I took a deep breath and began talking. The thing I recall most about her response was her annoyance about not being told before. She said I looked absolutely fine and recounted how many times she could have altered plans or helped me out physically — if only she had known. Her annoyance was short-lived and her honest desire to assist whenever I alerted her to it was very apparent. My hesitancy to reveal myself in an open, matter-of-fact way with a friend had cost me energy-time and had not allowed her to feel good about helping out. Being with me and helping whenever she could was more important than sharing certain activities.

What you tell someone is as important as how. Be direct when you need assistance or decline an invitation. Clarity leaves no room for confusion. Afford your friend or partner the opportunity to question you, alter plans and offer assistance. Do not misinterpret understanding and sympathy with pity. A well-intentioned question, change of plans, or helping hand will benefit everyone.

For many weeks my elderly neighbor was marketing with her new friend but always came home exhausted. She finally told me that she was going to have to start declining and was afraid she would lose her friendship. It turned out that her friend did not know of her pulmonary and fatigue problem and would park her car in a spot far away from the store entrance. She would also run other errands afterward. I suggested she be honest with her friend. Now, she gladly drops my neighbor at the market entrance before parking the car. Before picking her up she finds out if she is "up to" other errands. If not, she arranges her errands in such a way that dropping my neighbor back home is on the way to her next stop. Instead of being alone, they have each other and the open understanding they have has enriched their friendship.

It may be much easier to explain limits when you are older. Many times such a conversation will offer someone else the chance to say "me too!" But not all of us are retirees. Explaining to a co-worker, boss or peer may be more uncomfortable and difficult, but it is in your best interest. True friends do and feel better if they know. Honesty with your co-workers and boss leaves no room for accusations or recriminations later on.

The young woman in our first vignette must balance the demands of an illness with work and home. Reality tells her that to attend the business dinner would be detrimental to her health. But does she have to decline?

CONTROL THROUGH COMPROMISE AND READJUSTMENT

You can do things differently to allow for unexpected events by readjusting certain routines and compromising. Wake up later that particular morning. If this means changing the time of a scheduled activity, do so. Eliminate the chore from that day or swap it with one requiring less energy.

Save your personal hygiene for mid-afternoon.

Take a nap and eat small snacks throughout the day.

Do not fast, especially on a day with an extra event. Fasting uses immense amounts of metabolic energy.

SPREAD SOCIALIZING THROUGHOUT THE WEEK

Opt for the most enjoyment you can get from an event. This generally means looking at the energy needed for a given day in perspective to the whole week. Fewer extracurricular activities can mean you have more energy to enjoy leisure activities. Suggest ending times or go home and relax with your companions.

The retired couple in our second vignette maintains active lives and friendships. This does not mean, however, that they easily manage the dilemma of low energy. Decisions and choices have to be made so both will enjoy as much of each week as possible. There are always options. For instance, this couple could offer their bowling team the alternative of a closer restaurant. It would mean making the new arrangements themselves, but with much less effort than bowling and driving a long distance. They could enjoy both events without the disappointment of having to choose between the two.

Another alternative would be to offer light snacks at their home after bowling. The preparation could be spread out over the week and worked on together. If home is a retirement community or condominium, there is usually a recreation hall or room that can be used. If this is not possible, and your home is too small to handle a crowd, try extending invitations to individuals and couples on the team over a few weeks. This will allow sharing of good times with the added advantage of better energy-pacing.

A condominium neighbor of mine plays bridge every week at the senior center. If she finds she is not quite up to it, she arranges for a game to be played at her place on another day. There is never lack of a "fourth" — no matter what the day. Each person brings a "munchie" and a good time is had by all.

When I was a young child I wanted to participate in every trip my class went on and to take gym. It was imperative for me not to exert myself physically, so without my knowledge, my parents and teachers would create experiences for me during each trip. If there was a nature hike, I was part of a pond-study or rock-hound group. In gym, I was a referee or scorekeeper for those activities too strenuous. As I became older I realized my own limitations, but was never hindered by the thought that an alternative could not be found.

If your spouse or parent is in the hospital or nursing home, special considerations must be taken in order to provide them with positive socializing. Do not try to be the sole source for leisure and entertainment. Short visits from friends and other family members can provide you with time off. Make arrangements for a surprise visitor or special treat. Bring a loved pet to visit, with permission. Many agencies are realizing the value of pets in both recovery and socialization of the infirm and disabled.

Be productive during your visiting times. Do your bills, write some letters, read out loud or do some lap-stitchery. You cannot stare at each other all day, every day, without frustrations mounting. Interspersing some of your own, personal chores and enjoyments with your visit will help. It also provides for rests during a visit.

DO NOT ISOLATE YOURSELF

To suddenly find yourself alone, and perhaps in an alien environment, can lead to isolation. In our third vignette the woman is realistically assessing the present. The goal, however, is to make sure the hours do not drag. Today there are many community offerings for seniors and the general public. You just have to seek them out.

A good place to start is with your town hall. The annual report of any town or city will contain listings of all town departments. The office of community development, or the mayor's secretary, can give you listings as well. Other resources to tap are:

The local library. Ask to see the reference or head librarian.

The YMCA or YWCA.

Senior centers.

Area churches and synagogues. Many have community and social activities.

The telephone book yellow pages.

Your state's departments of education, employment & training, rehabilitation commission, or social services. These numbers can be found in the telephone book white pages under your state's name.

Local high schools for adult education classes and offerings.

Local colleges.

Departments of public transportation can give you vital information on transportation options and schedules.

The foster grandparent program or a senior pen-pal program through the school system can be rewarding experiences. It will keep you rejuvenated and put you in contact with other people in your community. The value for the child is immeasurable.

My son had a senior pen-pal in elementary school and fostered a relationship that has carried through to this day. It was also a great way to improve his handwriting and composition skills.

Anyone can withdraw or feel apart from life, not just the elderly. This is especially true if you have special limitations. The same resources can be tapped by all. Movement of mind and body toward something enjoyable or productive is what is important. Physical, intimate withdrawal is another form of isolation. Sexuality is communication, not just genital stimulation and intercourse. Sexuality exists throughout life but can be affected by factors such as age, physical limitations, decreased energy, pain, illness, pharmaceuticals, menopause, lack of a partner, fear, or residence in nursing homes and long-term care establishments. It is important to realize, however, that sexual expression not only means intimacy, but comfort and human contact.

CANDID COMMUNICATION IS VITAL

Sexual well-being is dependent on candid communication and your ability to adapt and adjust. Focus on the possibilities, not on what has been lost. Expression of love and caring does not have any limits or rules. The more candid you can be with your partner and yourself, the better. However, how to talk to your partner about your concerns, problems and desires can be difficult. Do not assume that you should be able to discuss intimate matters easily. Age, differing values and moralities, self-esteem, modesty, guilt and socio-environmental pressures all play a role in sexual expression. You may be, or become, perfectly happy in your relationship without it leading to intercourse. The simple act of pleasuring, touching, cuddling and comforting may bring fulfillment. As long as you are communicating, the pitfalls can be avoided.

The couple in our fourth vignette is reacting to a new emptiness in their relationship. The physical illness, pain and fatigue brought about a change in their sexual expression. Without talking to each other about this change, the feelings of emptiness will probably continue or get worse. Feelings of estrangement can lead to marital problems, anxiety, depression, tension and a hypochondriac cycle.

Ways to bridge the estrangement and ease into communicating about intimacy are quite painless. Start by allowing time for quiet, pleasant conversation. Talk about a good book or program you saw on television. Share a special food tidbit your partner likes. The result from such conversations can foster a new closeness and rediscovery of each other. You re-establish human contact with a loved one and this is the first step toward renewing sexual expression. Sharing "secrets" and revelations will become easier, thus paving the way for more frank and open discussions about sexuality.

Try bringing yourself to offer the reading of this chapter to your partner. It could serve as a good ice-breaker and give you specific areas to focus on in a more dispassionate way. Personalizing the information can come later.

Planning ahead for sexual activity is another way of improving communication. Partners need to have the ability to ask whether today — or now — is all right. Living with schedules and individuals' life-styles and limitations drains physical energy. There are practical problems as well. You want to be able to optimize your intimacy, not be hassled by it.

Spontaneity does not have to be forfeited. Learn how to be informal about planning ahead. Checking in with each other during the day can key you into moods and energies. Just as partners develop a shorthand for communication about other aspects of their lives, you can develop a shorthand for intimate communication. Certain phrases or tones of voice will tip you off. Say something like, "...how about plan B tonight?" The ability to ask and the assurance that love will be constant, even if the original intent is not achieved, is worth striving for.

New relationships are delicate and finding ways to discuss issues of sexuality can be overwhelming. First foster general conversation. Learn to laugh and cry together. Have good times. If you are not comfortable talking about your sexuality concerns and anxieties, maybe you are not ready to embark upon physical intimacy and consummation.

BE FRANK ABOUT PHYSICAL REQUIREMENTS

For the person with low energy or other impairment, the ultimate step in candid conversation is to be frank about physical requirements. The physics of sexual expression must also be understood. People who love you do not want to cause you pain or make you sick, so old "tried and true" ways of sexual expression may have to be supplanted by new methods and alternatives. Maintaining, or discovering, your personal sexual fulfillment means mastering the art of adaptation and readjustment.

One of my patients unburdened her overwhelming problem. She was beginning to dread physical intimacy with her spouse because she had great difficulty breathing whenever they "made love." I suggested changing to a sitting position with pillows to comfortably support her, or a change to a large, soft chair. This news was not received very enthusiastically, so we discussed how to improve her ability to openly talk to her spouse. Within the month I had a phone call from a very happy woman stating "the pillows worked!"

Joint pain, no matter what the cause, is generally associated with low energy. Do not hurry your intimate encounters. Enjoy your moments together. The traditional intercourse position of the man-on-the-top may be an aggravator. Gradual experimentation will uncover a variety of positions and practices that are equally enjoyable — and less painful and energy-depleting. Do not place all-consuming importance on sexual performance. This will only increase anxiety, pain and fatigue.

Kegel exercises will improve muscle tone in the genital-rectal area. To do this you contract your pubic and rectal muscles as if you were holding back from urinating and defecating. Doing this several times a day, contracting 20 to 30 times, each time, will help.

Isometrically contracted arm muscles should be avoided, so choose sexual positions that do not require supporting yourself on your arms. Lying on the bottom, with your partner on top allows you to participate in intercourse without great energy expenditure and no arm weight-bearing.

So that neither partner exerts muscle to support weight, lie on your sides facing the same direction, one arm extended to rest your head on. Another way to achieve the same goal is to face each other, one leg of each partner crossing over the other's.

Limited joint motion decreases flexibility. To increase comfort, both partners can stand, with the woman bending over a table and her arms resting on a pillow. Rear, vaginal entry by the man is thus supported by the woman.

For the woman who is not able to straighten her hips, the man can kneel, legs slightly apart and facing his partner. The woman lies on her back and slides her hips down toward the man, her legs up and supported by his torso.

If a woman cannot bend her hips or straighten her knees, she can lie with her hips at the edge of the bed and legs hanging down with knees bent and slightly apart. Her partner can than kneel or stand in front of her and lean over.

Sometimes severity of illness or pain can lead to the inability to bend either hips or knees. If this is so for the woman, she can lie on her stomach, head and torso resting on a pillow and the bed. The man can thus achieve a rear-entry position by pulling her towards him until her hips are at the edge of the bed and his hands are holding and supporting her legs slightly above the knees, with himself between them.

If you are paralyzed, there are specific and well documented methods for sexual activity. Have your physician or vocational therapist direct you to agencies or professionals specializing in this. Most larger hospitals have this service available.

Other means can be employed to assist in the prevention of fatigue and pain. To increase joint mobility, a prescribed exercise program from a certified physical therapy department should be started. Joint pain and pressure is greatly alleviated by a waterbed.

Prior to sexual activity you can use heat, such as a hot shower, hot-water bottle or heating pad, to increase flexibility and comfort. Empty your bladder for more comfortable playfulness and physical, sexual expression. By setting aside a rest-period before and after intercourse, you go far in conserving energy and preventing fatigue. A simple change to the morning may mean greater enjoyment due to greater energy reserves. With physician permission, you can try taking aspirin before and after intercourse to decrease pain. Keep in mind that sore joints may be an annoyance and impediment to physical performance but the goal is to maintain or gain that loving contact and sex with a caring partner.

Medications used for the treatment of many ailments can decrease sexual desire or impede performance. For a list of drugs affecting both male and female sexuality, please refer to *Aging: The Health Care Challenge*, by C.B. Lewis published by F. A. Davis Company, of Philadelphia. Most importantly, talk with your pharmacist and physician.

Heart disease and post-cardiac arrest generally involve a great deal of fear. As the spouse in vignette number five expresses, any thought of intimacy following heart attack is paralyzing. There is the fear of dying or recurring chest pain when making love. Your memory tortures you and the increasing look of betrayal and anguish on your partner's face only drives you further into yourself.

MISCONCEPTION AND IGNORANCE ARE ENEMIES

Take hold of your fears and learn the difference between fact and fiction. Include your spouse or loved one. The energy spent on your anxieties and isolation is much more than the energy-cost for intimacy. The possibility of a heart attack during intercourse is very small. It approximates climbing one or two flights of stairs or driving a car. If you can do this, then you are ready to resume sexual activity. Four to five weeks post-coronary is the usual time frame, barring other complications. In the interim, participation in touching, stroking and sharing quiet times is possible and beneficial.

When you are ready to resume sexual activity of a more physical nature, start out by taking a less active role. If you are anxious or fatigued, postpone sexual activity. Extreme heat or cold should be avoided so that you will not use vital energy in maintaining body temperature. Humidity is a particular energy sapper. By using non-weight-bearing positions you do not tire as easily and foreplay will afford your heart the chance to warm up.

An acquaintance has let me in on a family motto derived after his mid-life heart attack: "Just give me a jump start and I'll purr like a kitten." He and his wife never participated in much pre-arousal play and stimulation. To overcome his post-cardiac fear of intercourse, his vocational rehabilitation counselor suggested foreplay. It has now become an enjoyable preamble to sexual consummation and enjoyed for itself.

Disfigurement makes it difficult to maintain a good body image and erodes self-confidence and self-esteem. The individual in our final vignette considers this tantamount to damaged goods. Intimacy between a couple is often the only way to demonstrate love and support in the face of disfigurement. It offers a sense of normalcy and acceptance.

Allow your partner the chance to grow accustomed to

your scars or devices right along with you. Do not hide. Shame has no place in a loving, intimate relationship. This is best achieved right from the start and there are many things you can do to regain or improve intimacy. Reassure your partner that you still find him or her sexually desirable.

Do a lot of touching and cuddling. When you walk by, a soft caress on the shoulder can be so comforting and loving.

Do not look away. If there is hesitancy in the beginning, start by using positions where you do not face each other and remain partially clothed. With time and loving, you will find you will not look away.

Be the instigator for a sexually arousing situation.

Sensually undress your partner.

Change appliances or dressings together.

Talk about each other's fears and concerns.

Be willing to experiment with different sexual positions.

Share fantasies.

Leave little handwritten notes of love and reassurance where your partner can find them during the day.

Once again, keeping the avenues of communication open means better understanding and fewer anxious moments.

ALTERNATE METHODS FOR SEXUAL ENJOYMENT

Alternatives exist to aid intercourse or as independent activities. Understandably, age and different socialization and value orientations may preclude the use of these methods. It is okay to avoid such alternatives, because, loving and sexuality are not dependent only upon intercourse and genital stimulation. The idea of ever using any device or alternate means for arousal so upset my elderly neighbor that it tied her up in knots for weeks. Her husband's doctor had told her to "do things" to her husband that revolted her. She also felt, because of her religion, that she would be doing something sinful. After a tearful visit it became clear to me that the physician had not taken the time to explain that the importance was to maintain their warm and loving relationship. The methods were not the issue. Had he simply directed her to touch, cuddle and be supportive, she could have taken it from there, using methods comfortable to them as a couple.

If stimulation and maintaining sexual excitement is a problem, methods of more direct genital contact can be used. This includes fondling and rhythmic stroking of the genitalia for maintenance of an erection or stimulating vaginal lubrication. To greatly reduce the risk of over exertion, oral stimulation of genitals and self or mutual masturbation can take the place of intercourse — or serve as a prelude. It may even be preferred, especially if physical limitations exist. A vibrator can be used if there is peripheral muscle weakness in the hands. Strapping it to the hand prevents slipping. A vibrator is also an alternative when you just cannot expend any extra energy. Penile prostheses are available through physicians specializing in impotence and a hard, doughnut-shaped device made of rubber can be used to assist in maintaining erections.

The pleasure and therapeutic value of massage is becoming increasingly popular and accepted. It aids in relaxation of muscles and can decrease pain. It increases circulation, helps prevent swelling and increases mobility. Sometimes we cannot achieve sexual fulfillment without the assistance of professionals. There are many rehabilitation groups and settings offered for just such help and support. Most larger hospitals and universities have departments dedicated to sexuality counseling and rehabilitation. Social service and vocational rehabilitation departments are great resources for referral and information. Begin by talking with your doctor, who may not be aware that you have these concerns.

DESIRE AND OPPORTUNITY
DO NOT ALWAYS COINCIDE

The reality of life is that we may not always have a special person with whom to share our desires — sexual or not. Opportunity and interest do not always coincide. Among the elderly population statistics show women outnumber men by almost four to one; and with the rate of divorce being what it is, as well as AIDS, opportunity may be quite elusive.

There is social pressure, although slowly changing, to discourage elder adults from seeking new relationships with sexual overtones. Most often this occurs between widows and widowers and their children. We still tend to associate sexual attraction with the young body and feel embarrassed trying to see our parent as "sexy." If the elders are viewed as sexually nonfunctional, they will often fulfill this expectation. The options of maintaining sexuality through masturbation or homosexuality are not actively pursued because age, familial and social pressures and prejudices tend to eliminate them from consideration.

Any person should be given the chance to pursue changing patterns of practice without retribution, especially from loved ones or friends. These private matters are for them to deal with as individuals. Be supportive and caring.

Nursing homes and long-term care facilities face the problem of the sexually isolated person as well. It is often forgotten that there is great healing power in being held, touched and caressed and for people living in these environments, there is generally no opportunity for such expression. Speak to personnel about the possibility of an overnight guest. See if privacy can be assured without locking doors.

If you are alone and experiencing all those desires that are very much a part of life, there are ways to maintain a good self-image and keep depression and anxiety at bay. Try self-stroking, caressing or masturbation to reaffirm that you have not lost your desire or ability to feel and respond like a sexual being.

By keeping yourself mentally and physically fit within the bounds of your energy, you will have the positive outlook needed to deal with anything, including being alone.

BE A THINKING PERSON AND PROTECT

Before concluding this chapter it is important to briefly mention the importance of protection from unwanted pregnancy and disease. Sexuality and sexual activity are integral to life. While you are striving for maintenance or recovery of this part of your life, you must also think of potential outcomes. Unwanted or life-threatening pregnancies and sexually transmitted diseases can happen, but they can be prevented as well. Use one or more of the available methods of birth control if you are sexually active. Even if certain methods are not part of your religious beliefs, there is generally one that is acceptable. To know what is available and best for you, start with your doctor, family planning clinic or public health office. This is one area in which you want to be a thinking person because your health and energy can be devastatingly affected.

LEISURE AND PLAY WILL REAP REWARDS

We have discussed how important it is to build leisure and fun into your everyday life. It is not always easy and many things factor into how successful you can be. However, there is always an alternative and fulfillment is around-the-corner. You must be willing to readjust your thinking and behaviors and not dwell on the impossibles. Communicate on all levels and you will have found the key.

Making It "Work" — 7

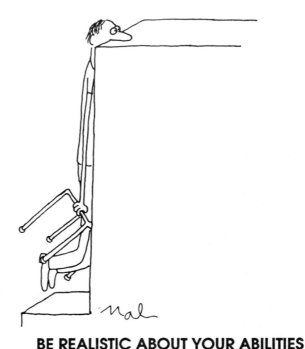

**BE REALISTIC ABOUT YOUR ABILITIES
AND LIMITATIONS**

**DENIAL LEADS TO FATIGUE
AND DISAPPOINTMENT**

**BEWARE OF CLIMATE DEMANDS ON
YOUR ENERGY RESERVE**

PLAN REST PERIODS

JOB CONSIDERATIONS

For the person with low energy or disability, career choice and considerations are extremely important in maintaining quality of life. A hastily made choice, or persistence in a non-suitable job, can spell energy disaster and lead to illness.

BE REALISTIC ABOUT YOUR ABILITIES AND LIMITATIONS

To make a career choice or change, take a good look at your present self and ask some important questions. Be brutally honest about your answers, because people in the work force will be.

Are you academically or technically able to do the job?

Does this decision reflect a change in your health and physical state? If so, what has changed?

What are your physical capabilities and limitations? List them, starting from the head and working on down to your toes.

Know your energy limits and list them.

What are other obligations that will be energy draining?

Is transportation an issue?

Do you need health care insurance?

Is diet a consideration?

Do you have a caring, support system in place?

Are you the sole provider and what if you lose your job?

Are others dependent upon your income and health?

Is the dollar value earned more than the energy exerted to carry out your job?

When making career choices the central issue is the physical demands of the work. Perhaps the job was perfect, when you first started but ten years have passed and your energy levels are much lower. Even if you have been incapacitated you may be tempted to return to a job you cannot feasibly perform because of your need for income and health insurance.

DENIAL LEADS TO FATIGUE AND DISAPPOINTMENT

If you are going to deny the realities of the physical demands of your job, then fatigue will be a constant companion and you will face many disappointing choices when you have to give up an activity or task you had planned on doing. A worse-case-scenario is being let go because you cannot perform your job.

A young man shut himself in his room for days, extremely depressed and non-communicative. It was only after his mother received a phone call from the payroll office at work that the family learned he had been fired. Recent flare-ups of his rheumatoid arthritis meant increased joint pain and exhaustion with little exertion. He kept quiet and over the month let his duties slide. Without any knowledge of why, even upon direct questioning, his boss had no choice but to fire him. His particular job required a lot of physical effort and it was vital that each worker do his share to meet production goals. It was a sad time for all.

Had this young man honestly assessed the job's physical demands and not denied his limits, he could have approached his boss to inquire about temporary reassignment or a short leave with pay. His denial not only led to exhaustion and pain, but to disappointment and upset as well. There was certainly no attention paid to energy conservation.

BEWARE OF CLIMATE DEMANDS ON YOUR ENERGY RESERVE

It is well documented that the environment plays a role in how we are able to function and carry out various tasks. In the workplace this plays a key role in how well you can conserve energy.

Extremes of temperature require the use of more metabolic energy to maintain normal body temperature. When accompanied by humid or arid conditions, more energy is called for. To the person battling decreased energy, this can spell trouble.

Particular jobs may require you to work in extremes of temperatures. Some examples are:

Butcher
Construction worker
Florist
Letter carrier
Archaeologist
Field biologist
Operating room technician
Computer systems operator
Commercial laundry
Fuel station attendant

House painter

Carpenter

If you work indoors, make sure that the heating and air-conditioning systems work and that there is proper and adequate ventilation. Do not hesitate to be a squeaky wheel if these systems are not functioning properly. If there are large windows, shades or blinds can help to either keep the cold out or heat in. They are also sources of additional ventilation. Ceiling fans can reduce heat loss by circulating the hot air that rises, and when air-conditioning is used, they can actually cut costs substantially due to movement of air. The temperature does not have to be kept as cold.

Dressing in layers is always a good idea, for you are always prepared — cold or hot. This also affords you the chance to go from casual to dressy or business-like. Warm or cold feet can make a difference, so wear outfits that will accommodate the particular indoor environment you work in.

A co-worker keeps a pair of warm wool socks and ballet leg-warmers in her bottom desk drawer for those particularly drafty days.

My grandmother took great pride in knitting me a neutral-colored sweater to keep in the office for when it gets chilly. It matches anything I choose to wear and reminds me of her when I put it on. Double the warmth in one!

A cotton "dickie" can provide that extra neck warmth whenever necessary.

Take water along to maintain hydration, which is very important for constant body temperature and energy saving.

CONSIDER TEMPORARY
OR PART-TIME EMPLOYMENT

Temporary or part-time employment can provide you with that necessary transition to full-time work. If full-time is not for you, then temporary or part-time employment may be the answer. It can also provide you with the flexibility to search for practical alternatives while earning money. Actively seek out the proper employment for yourself. Read the newspaper and network. Networking is making contacts with various individuals in various job settings, whether or not there currently is employment opportunity. Keep a file and routinely call them. Many companies, industries, healthcare providers and universities post job openings on employee bulletin boards. Make it part of your plan to routinely visit those you are interested in because often jobs are first posted internally and then advertised.

The phone can be your best advocate and energy saver, so use it whenever possible. Save yourself those wasted trips to gather information. Have information and even applications mailed. Find out before hand what documentation you need to take with you to an interview.

VOLUNTEER WORK AFFORDS FLEXIBILITY

If a routine, daily work schedule is not practical, you can volunteer. Volunteer jobs can be fulfilling work experiences and you generally can pick and choose your days and hours. Rigid time requirements are not part of most volunteer positions, so this fits the energy-poor individual very well.

You can choose from many different volunteer programs. There is almost one to fit every person's interest. There are many national volunteer programs and you can find out about them by calling your state capital. The 800 telephone directory service can also be a good resource.

Most cities and towns have volunteer programs. Call the town hall and they will direct you to the person in charge. The library will carry directories of volunteerism or they will maintain files in their reference section. Speak with the reference or head librarian for these materials. Almost all hospitals, universities and public school systems have volunteer programs. Call these institutions to be directed to the appropriate person. Churches and synagogues also do volunteer work and the office secretary can tell you who to talk with.

SPECIFIC JOBS REQUIRE SPECIFIC CONSIDERATIONS

When you get a job, there are specifics to consider before signing your name on that dotted line.

For anyone with disability, low-energy or who is close to retirement, the primary concern should be the all-important benefit package. It behooves you to take home less dollars, if it means full and employer-paid benefits. When choosing between two jobs, it will be tempting to take the one with higher salary, but look closely at the benefits offered.

Ask someone to explain the benefits in detail before you agree to take the position. Do not let an employer tell you that you cannot take the information packet home with you to study. Do not be surprised if you have to have someone explain the information to you several times. Benefit information is complex, so take your time. It is well worth the effort.

When considering a job, think carefully about the hours. Rigid hours with no flexibility can be a problem for the person with low energy. Some places of business offer mother's hours, job-sharing, staggered shifts and four or five day weeks. Employers are also making it possible to work split hours. This means you work for a few hours, leave and then come back for the remainder of your day's time.

A young woman just starting out in a new job assumed that the hours she was given were set. What she had not been told was that staggered hours were possible. She found out about it at lunch when some co-workers were discussing their end-of-shift times. As soon as she could, she made an appointment with her supervisor and was able to start two hours earlier in the morning — when she had the most energy and was at her best.

Make sure that your energy needs can meet the hour requirements of your job. Be frank with your superiors about your special concerns and needs. Many times personalized arrangements can be made.

PHYSICAL LAYOUT IS IMPORTANT

You may have to travel between offices and departments if your job is in a large company. Think about whether you have the stamina for it. Check if there are conveyor, tube or messenger systems to deliver materials. If there are elevators or escalators you will be able to conserve your energies. Sometimes travel between buildings is necessary, so consider if this will pose a problem. Wheelchairs and crutches need special access and facilities. Make sure they are available.

Accessible restrooms are notorious for being tucked out-of-the-way in older buildings. Locate your work area and scout ahead.

In our car society we tend to forget the value of mass transportation. The ability to be "driven" to work because your job is on a bus or commuter route is terrific. You can rest easy knowing that you have back-up in case your car breaks down, or you can elect to use this alternate means of travel on a regular basis.

If you drive to work, locate the parking facilities ahead of time. This will help you to know and plan for the expected energy expenditure of walking to and from the lot. Handicapped parking spaces are mandatory in most states. If there are of marked spaces — use them.

PLAN REST PERIODS

Fatigue has been discussed in previous chapters and many of the techniques and planning used to avoid tiring situations can be carried over into the workplace. You ask, "rest at work?" Yes!

Start by knowing the physical and energy-draining obstacles you will face daily and then brainstorm for solutions. If furniture you use is uncomfortable and taxing, find out if substitutes are available. You should be able to relax in your work furniture as well as be productive.

The desk height in my first office was quite high and very uncomfortable for my four foot eleven inches. By morning's end my shoulders ached from the exertion of leaning up and over to write and type and my feet were numb because they barely touched the floor. I scouted around and found that there was an empty computer desk which is lower in height. You can bet that I had one of the janitors help me swap. I brought from home an old, low footstool. Presto, no more shoulder aches and muscle fatigue.

Most workplaces have a lounge for breaks. Instead of the traditional two, fifteen minute breaks, ask if it is possible to take them as five minute breaks throughout the day. You can sit and do relaxation techniques at your post; sometimes you can get up and stretch. Passive desk exercises will rejuvenate tense, stiff, tired muscles. No matter what the temptation, do not work through lunch. You need the nourishment for maintenance of metabolic energy and physical stamina. Try and get some fresh air during this time as well. If the lunchroom is too raucous for you, try a lounge or search out a quiet corner. The normal stresses and noise of the routine work day do not have to carry over into your lunch break. An employer may be more than happy to have you take a short lunch-nap somewhere private, such as the nurses' or infirmary office — especially if it means continued productivity for the balance of the day. Building in these rest periods will be a deterrent to exhaustion.

BACK-UP AVAILABILITY
ASSURES THE JOB GETS DONE

It is unwise for anyone with energy problems or disability to have a job and be solely responsible for producing an end product. This can lead to employer frustration and anger, if in the middle of a job you just cannot go on due to your limitations. Degree of fatigue on a given day is unpredictable. If you can call on someone to step in as substitute when you cannot continue, or even go to work, then the job is accomplished and everyone is happy. Your willingness to honor and uphold your responsibilities earns respect from both superiors and co-workers and makes you feel good in the process. You do not have to exert energy on worrying about the job getting done or if this wrinkle will cost you your job.

BE UP-FRONT ABOUT YOUR CONDITION

You live with your condition daily, so it becomes second nature to you. Often it is easy to forget that not everyone understands it. Our combined work and personal experiences have shown that honesty with an employer — from the start — serves you best. How many times we were asked whether a particular disease or disability should be noted on the application form! For good reason people fear revealing health information because of discrimination and prejudice. But disability has come into its time. Employers are much more willing to accommodate someone's limitations. They are often mandated by law to do so.

The federal government has passed The Americans With Disabilities Act (ADA). This Act is on equal footing with the Civil Rights Act. It will, at the least, guarantee anyone with a disability the mechanism for legally pursuing and obtaining rights denied them. Your state senator's office will have copies of this law.

Have frank discussions with your superiors, alert and work with the health office and educate with facts to dispel misconceptions. The time spent is well spent. Greater understanding means more interpersonal and professional support from colleagues and administration. It also means a more satisfying and happy work situation for you.

Running
The Marathon — 8

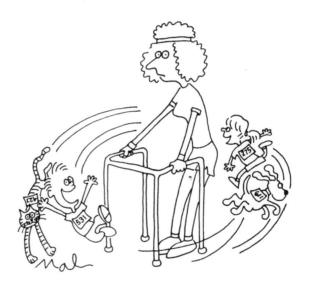

INFANCY: SLEEP WHEN THE BABY SLEEPS

TODDLERHOOD: THOROUGHLY CHILDPROOF YOUR HOUSE

GIVE YOURSELF A BREAK

SCHOOL AGE CHILDREN: ADJUST YOUR SCHEDULE

PARENTING

Child care is exhausting work; it is also one of life's most rewarding experiences. Many disabled and chronically ill people are parents or hope to be some day. Many elderly people are grandparents. For those with low energy levels, taking an active part in raising a child is like running the marathon — every day!

When you and your spouse are making decisions about having children or about how to share the child care responsibilities, be brutally honest with yourselves about your abilities. There is no place here for false optimism. Taking care of a baby or young child is very demanding.

Grandparents with low energy levels should be very cautious about babysitting. Be wise and remember that the safety of your grandchild is the most important consideration.

In this chapter we will present many energy conservation techniques to use in parenting. We hope they will make your task less hard; but they will not make it easy. As parents we know the joys children bring. We know, too, the incredible energy costs involved in caring for them.

A pregnant woman in a wheelchair prepared for her new role by practicing child care with a doll. When she tried her new skills on a friend's six-month-old, however, the woman found that the baby was too heavy for her to lift. She held the baby comfortably when he was quiet, but did not feel safe when he started squirming. The woman was disappointed; but the experience helped her plan realistically for the care of her child.

DELEGATION IS A KEY TO
ENERGY CONSERVATION

Delegation is never easy and the birth of a child often complicates it. The intricate balance of family responsibilities collapses when a baby arrives. Roles are suddenly shifted and challenged as parents become grandparents, wife becomes a mother, and husband becomes a father. Babysitters suddenly play crucial parts in the family structure. Delegation becomes an energy draining task in itself when it entails interviewing sitters, coordinating schedules, and anticipating baby's needs. Use diplomacy and planning when arranging for help with your child and have back-up plans for days when the babysitter gets sick, your spouse is late, or you do not feel well.

There are many tasks involved in the daily care of a child. When you parcel them out, save some playtime for yourself. Do not exhaust yourself with caretaker chores while someone else plays with the child. Hand off more of the work and leave yourself the energy for playing, talking, and cuddling.

INFANCY: SLEEP WHEN THE BABY SLEEPS

Infants sleep a lot — but not for long periods and, too often, not at night. The only way for a new parent to cope is to adapt to the baby's rhythm as much as possible. Cut all your other responsibilities back to the absolute essentials for a while and enjoy this crazy but precious time with your newborn.

Parent and baby can spend the whole day in bed together. With diaper changing supplies next to the bed and a few toys, you can play, snuggle and sleep together. Nursing mothers will find lying down the least tiring position for feeding. Whether bottle or breast feeding, the bed pillows can be arranged to get parent and baby in comfortable positions.

For transporting the baby, you may want a carrier pouch. These enable the parent to use good body mechanics by having the weight of the baby close to the adult's body. Arms do not tire from holding the baby and are free to do other things. Many families only use a stroller for the baby outdoors. Bring it inside and wheel the baby from room to room. A reclining back makes it a portable bed for the infant as well.

The floor is a very safe place for the baby — there is nowhere to fall! Changing, playing, and sleeping can all be done on a quilt or blanket spread on the floor. Just make sure that you get down there to interact eye-to-eye with your little one.

Some baby supplies are energy savers: premixed formula, disposable diapers, and premoistened wipes. To simplify dressing the baby, look for front closures and roomy sizes. Set up several changing stations around the house (especially in two story homes). Change the baby on the floor, your lap or someplace you can sit down and the baby is protected from rolling off. Adjust the crib mattress to a comfortable height for you to avoid unnecessary bending and lifting.

New parents need to make use of every energy conservation technique. Be creative in problem solving and apply the principles of work simplification until you and baby find what works for you.

While in the hospital or birthing center, discuss your

concerns about low-energy parenthood with the staff. The obstetrical nurses or midwives can educate you about the care of your newborn and give advice about your special circumstances.

Nurse with the baby on a pillow on your lap or on a wheelchair tray.

Modify a carrier for nursing.

Place the child in an infant seat for feeding.

Get into the tub with baby for bathing to avoid bending and lifting.

Use more sponge baths for baby.

Line the sink with a towel and bathe baby there.

Attach a wide safety strap with VELCRO™ closure to the changing table for security.

Keep a hamper or laundry bag at each changing station.

Stock up on pillow cases and waterproof pads. Lay a pad and then a pillowcase on top of the crib sheet so when baby spits up or wets you do not have to change the sheets, just replace the pillowcase and liner.

Use an intercom.

Bottles of premixed formula can be kept at the bedside. Types that require refrigeration can be stored in a cooler.

TODDLERHOOD: CHILDPROOF YOUR HOUSE

When your child becomes mobile it is essential that you childproof the environment. Making your home safe for a toddler will not only give you peace of mind, it will save your energy. You will be spared jumping up to pull baby's hand away from an electric outlet or diving to catch a falling lamp. Even a sluggish toddler can get into mischief with lightning speed. Prepare for it.

Childproofing a home involves removing all potential dangers. All cleaning supplies and medicines need to be stored in high, latched cabinets. Remove breakables or move them out of reach. Electric outlets need to be covered and electric cords made inaccessible. Coffee tables with sharp edges should be padded. Gate off stairs. Put latches on kitchen and bathroom cabinets and drawers. Barricade woodstoves and fireplaces. Beyond these general guidelines, you will need to check your house for its particular dangers. You can do this by getting down on your hands and knees and crawling around. Looking at the world from baby's level will help you spot hazards.

As a low-energy parent, you will want a place to spend the day with your toddler. The bed is no longer a safe or stimulating play space. Baby is ready for action in a space without hard edges. Now the two of you need a "padded" room! Prepare a room in your home with all the essentials you and your child will need for the day. Close the door or gate it off from the rest of the house. This room should be thoroughly childproofed so baby can play safely — even tossing balls and riding scooters. You will want a sofa or recliner so you can stretch out sometimes. Equip the room with toys for baby, of course, but also with activities for yourself. While you spend the day with your child you could fold yesterday's laundry, pay the bills, read, do handwork, listen to the radio, watch television or write the grocery list. By adding a telephone and note pad, this room can become a control center. You may want to stock the room with snack foods for the baby and a blanket for naps. Keeping up with a toddler takes a lot of energy. A "padded" room confines the child while providing a safe, stimulating environment for both of you.

If you do not have a room you can dedicate to baby in your house or apartment, a playpen may meet your needs. Choose a well-made one with soft sides. A playpen on wheels permits you to move baby from room to room with you.

TODDLERS AND PRESCHOOLERS: CONSISTENT DISCIPLINE AND INDEPENDENCE TRAINING HAVE LONGTERM PAYOFFS

By thoroughly childproofing your house, you have eliminated much of the need for verbally restraining your child. Still occasions arise when a parent has to say, "no." When you do, be firm and follow through. Consistent discipline is very important. When your child is old enough to run, you may not be able to catch up. You need to know that when you yell, "Stop!" the child will freeze. Being consistent in disciplining is not always easy and it is energy consuming, but a parent with low energy has to do it. You have to train your child to respond to your voice because you may not always be able to move swiftly enough to intervene physically.

Independence training should start early in your family also. Very young children can learn to dress themselves, make their beds, and pick up toys. At first they do these jobs very slowly and badly; but be patient and teach them again. Family members are more interdependent when one has low energy. Young children can be taught to do more by themselves and to help others. In the process they increase their self-esteem and learn to be thoughtful and considerate of others.

GIVE YOURSELF A BREAK

Parents need respite from child care. The care of toddlers and preschoolers is less physically demanding than that of infants, but more emotionally taxing. Children of this age want a lot of attention. They have great curiosity, increasing needs for socializing, and short attention spans. Children test the limits of their world, often pushing the limits of their parents' patience in the process. Thankfully they sleep longer at night; but they nap less during the day. Parenting children of this age is a lot of fun and a lot of hard work. Plan to take breaks from it.

One free and easy way to schedule breaks is to find another parent and take turns caring for each other's children. Your "padded" room could surely accommodate another child for a while and in return you can look forward to some time to yourself. Parents often find that a day with a visiting playmate is somewhat easier as the two children entertain each other.

Babysitters are another option. A babysitter in the evening or on the weekend can give you and your spouse a chance to spend some time together, even if it is just to go out for a drive or a cup of coffee. You do not need to spend the money on a restaurant meal to enjoy some time together.

One mother has a babysitter come every afternoon for 45 minutes so she can pick up her husband after work. The couple enjoys the quiet time to talk together before the commotion of the family dinner hour.

Babysitters can also be used while you stay at home. Perhaps you can find a teenager or even a preteen to come over after school and play with your child while you retreat to the bedroom. We know many parents who have done this. Some use the time for a hobby such as sewing or refinishing furniture that they cannot do safely with children nearby. Some use a sitter in order to prepare for entertaining. Others simply want the time to have a shower and a nap. This inhouse arrangement is a nice way to begin training a preteen to become a full-fledged babysitter for you in the future. Kids of intermediate age are often thrilled to have a first job and make very good playmates for younger children.

By the time your child is two-and-a-half or three years old you can consider a nursery school of some kind. The offerings and prices vary from community to community. Ask other parents for recommendations and use the telephone to explore this option. In some towns, popular nursery schools fill up early so begin asking around long before you are ready to send your child. Preschools give your child a social experience while giving you a break.

Choose a high chair with a one-handed tray release mechanism, a seat belt, and a raised edge around the tray.

A feeding table is an alternative to a high chair. It is lower and more stable than a high chair and therefore safer for very energetic children who might squirm free of the high chair seatbelt.

Older and younger children can bathe together and help each other wash.

A child can be more independent dressing if the clothes are generous in size and pull-on styles. Shoes with VELCRO™ closures are easy to manage.

Tethers of various kinds help parents keep track of fleet footed toddlers when walking together.

Prepare an outdoor play yard like the "padded" room. Enclose and babyproof the space.

Teach preschoolers to use a hand-held vacuum to clean up crumbs after a meal.

SCHOOL AGE CHILDREN: ADJUST YOUR SCHEDULE

When children begin school, parents find that the routine and pacing of their day has to be adjusted to match the school day. Households typically have an hour of great activity in the morning. Before school there is a flurry of dressing, eating breakfast and the gathering of lunch boxes, school bags, homework, permission slips and so on. After the children leave for school the house is quiet — until mid afternoon. The late afternoon and evening are busy with play dates, scout meetings, lessons, homework and baths. Low energy parents have to adjust their personal routines in order to have energy for parenting early in the morning and late in the day. For working parents this may be difficult. If you have the flexibility, however, you would be wise to plan your day differently now in order to have stamina for the evening. Perhaps you can get up earlier in the morning to do your personal care before the children awake. Alternatively, you could delay your personal care chores until after they have left for school. Perhaps you will need an afternoon nap to see you through the busy evening hours. School age children still need your care and attention; they just need it during different time periods.

Continue to encourage independence in your children. Children in the primary grades are capable of almost complete independence in personal care. By now they can bathe and shampoo alone. They can clear their dishes from the table after each meal. They should be able to fix themselves a simple, nutritious lunch. As they grow, so should their responsibilities. In time your children should be caring for their own rooms — dusting, vacuuming, changing the bed linens. Older children can take responsibility for their own laundry and should learn how to cook a meal for the family. Independence training teaches your children practical skills they will use for a lifetime and it teaches values of responsibility and family obligation.

Babysitters are still necessary at this stage, though you may find new ways of using them. You might like to use a sitter to watch siblings while you take one child out for some special time together. You may want to hire a preteen or teenager to teach your child to ride a bike or to supervise at the playground. Some parents take a sitter along on vacation to lend a hand at the beach or amusement park. Delegating is an important tool for saving energy.

Choose clothes for school the night before to cut down on the morning rush.

Make lunches the night before.

Carpool.

Do not use bedspreads, just a blanket or comforter that

a child can pull up and smooth out.

Train young children to put dirty clothes in the hamper as soon as they remove them.

Young children can learn to strip sheets off a bed, set the table, and feed pets.

Feather dusters are very appealing. Children like to dust with them.

Try to schedule your errands on quieter days. Don't tire yourself grocery shopping on a day when its your turn to drive the carpool to soccer practice.

Look for sensible ways you can help out at school. Do not volunteer to chaperone the field trip. Do offer to make telephone calls for the parents association when necessary.

Children are active, impulsive, noisy creatures and that's healthy. We hope the energy conservation techniques suggested in this chapter will help you enjoy the time with your special children because, whether you are a parent, grandparent, aunt, uncle, or friend, children can add a unique and precious element to your life.

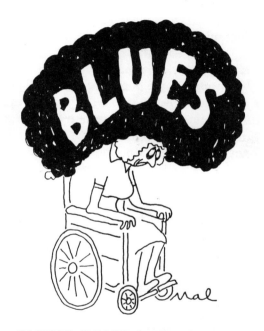

TAKING CONTROL SAVES ENERGY
**IDENTIFY YOUR PERSONAL SUPPORTS,
AND USE THEM**
LEARN HOW TO RELAX
FIND A SUPPORT GROUP

EMOTIONS

My husband and I used to be partners. Then came my stroke and suddenly I was totally dependent on him. I lost my sense of control, my independence. That was very hard to adjust to — harder than the physical problems.

There are so many things I want to do but I can't. I feel jealous of my friends; but mostly I feel angry.

I feel like I have a high energy personality trapped inside a low energy body. It's so frustrating.

Sometimes I just feel so sorry for myself I cry.

I say to myself, "C'mon. No pain, no gain." See, I've always been an athlete — strong, tough — so I push myself to keep going. But then I pay for it. I get wiped out and sick. I feel mad at myself and defeated.

I used to run this household. Everyone in the family relied on me. Now I can't do it all. My self-esteem is gone. I'm depressed.

Individuals react to low energy levels with a variety of different emotions; but in every case low energy exacts a psychological toll. The emotional component which accompanies a loss of energy often complicates one's adjustment to it. In previous chapters we have presented methods of work simplification and principles of energy conservation to help you cope with your compromised physical condition. In this chapter we urge you to attend to your psychological condition because the two are so intimately entwined.

It is natural and reasonable to feel down about a lack of energy. The catch is that experiencing the emotions further drains your energy reserves. Emotions make energy demands on your body and when you are already struggling to get through the physical challenges of the day, their toll is serious. Ignoring your feelings is not the solution. Alcohol and drugs are not the answer. You need to acknowledge the emotions you are experiencing and address them head on, just as you do your physical limitations.

BUDGET ENERGY FOR EMOTIONS

If you are the disciplined type you can budget time (and energy) to devote to emotions. For an allotted amount of time you dwell on the anger, discouragement, frustration, or jealousy you feel. When the time is up you get on with business. Obviously this will not work for everyone, but as planning and scheduling become routine you may find that making appointments with your psyche follows naturally.

Diane mentioned in a lecture that she devotes 50 minutes a week to feeling sorry for herself.

"Why 50 minutes?" she was asked. "How did you arrive at that amount of time?"

"I started that when I was first working. The weekends were no problem, but the weekdays were rough so I allotted 10 minutes a day to self-pity. Over the years I've stayed with that original 50 minutes a week."

TAKING CONTROL SAVES ENERGY

What situations do you find stressful? What causes you to worry or feel nervous? By identifying the kinds of events or circumstances that make you anxious, you can prepare for them.

If a telephone conversation with a particular friend or relative always leaves you feeling spent, take control. You place the call to control the timing. Plan this energy expenditure as you would any other.

If watching news of wars and disasters upsets you, turn off the television. If talk shows get you steamed, change the station. Take control.

Good times are energy drains too. Before going to a gathering or holiday celebration, rest. Plan to take breaks away from the crowd during the affair. And be wise enough to leave before you *become* exhausted.

You do not have as much energy as your peers or as you yourself once did. Recognize this fact and accept it as part of who you are now. Equally difficult, perhaps, is telling others that you cannot do certain things. Learn to say "no." Do not take on more than you can manage comfortably. It is essential to your physical and mental health. There are many things in life that we cannot change, that we must learn to accept. But by taking control of those things we can change, we can reduce the tension and stress in our lives.

IDENTIFY YOUR PERSONAL SUPPORTS, AND USE THEM.

Just as it is necessary to recognize the causes of stress in your life and to plan for them, it is important to identify the people and activities which make you happy and make time for them. Think about the people who make you laugh, the people who are good listeners, and those who give constructive advice. Find time — and energy — to spend with these people. Write a letter. Make a phone call. When you are feeling down, turn to a supportive friend and ask for help. Do not expect others to guess what you are feeling, no matter how close you are. Tell them.

What activities do you find relaxing? Which ones make you happy? What gives you a sense of satisfaction? Prioritize the activities in your day to allow time for some of the things you enjoy. You will be happier — and better company for others — if you make time for a favorite activity. When each day seems overwhelming, it may look impossible to find the energy for a leisure activity; but if you can let another task go undone and direct some energy to having fun, you will surely feel better.

Activities can also serve to work out tension. A soothing, rhythmic activity may help you cool down after a stressful event. A forceful, pounding activity can vent angry feelings. Making something — a gift, a meal, a card — for someone else can shift your emotional focus toward someone you care for and away from yourself.

LEARN HOW TO RELAX

The breaks you take during the day will not be beneficial unless you truly relax. Simply sitting or lying down will not restore your energy; you must clear your mind of worry also.

A business executive used to rest at his desk every day after lunch. He held his keys in his hand, leaned back in his chair and closed his eyes. When he was completely relaxed his keys would drop to the floor and wake him. He then felt refreshed and ready to resume work.

Perhaps, like the business executive, you have already developed a relaxation routine; if not, the following suggestions may be helpful. These methods work for us or for people we know. If you would like more information about relaxation, check the library and bookstore. There are many books, tapes, and even courses on these techniques.

Visualization helps many people relax. To visualize, daydream about a scene you find very restful. Some people return in their minds to a place they have been before; others imagine a setting of serenity. You may try several visualizations until you "find" a favorite place to return again and again. If you like the seashore, for instance, try to imagine sitting on one specific beach. Feel the warmth of the sun on your skin, the texture of the sand. Hear the rhythmic sound of the waves. Smell the salt air. By concentrating on a soothing scene, you forget for a while the concerns and anxieties of the day.

One client chose the seashore for her visualization. She was encouraged to imagine drifting in a small boat, rocking gently with the swells.

"It won't work," the client interrupted.

"Why not?"

"I get seasick!"

The seashore may not be your choice. Here are some other ideas to get you started:

Sit by a fireplace, watching the flames dance. Feel the warmth. Smell the wood smoke. Hear the crackle.

Ice skate on a pond frozen smooth as glass. Glide effortlessly around and around.

Sit on a hilltop, leaning against a sun-warmed rock and watch the sun set across the valley.

Music greatly affects our moods; it can be a powerful tool for relaxation. Choose music that you find calming. Prepare for a music break by positioning yourself comfortably and adjusting the volume down until the music is just loud enough to hear. Clear your mind of other thoughts and concentrate on the music. You might like to use music as a background for your visualization. Slow, soothing music can also be helpful when doing a difficult task; it can provide a rhythm for your movements and reduce your agitation.

Progressive relaxation techniques focus on relaxing muscle groups. Muscles held tense contribute to fatigue. Some people can "go limp" very readily, others need to learn how to relax their muscles. Begin progressive relaxation by reclining and closing your eyes. Concentrate first on your toes and feet. Tense every muscle in your feet and hold that tension for 10 seconds. (Do not hold your breath.) Then relax the muscles of your feet and toes. Relax them until your feet seem to be weightless. (Some people like to think of their limbs as becoming very heavy, rather than weightless, and sinking into the bed or chair.) Next move up to the muscles of your legs. Tense, hold, relax. Progress through your buttocks and abdomen, torso, hands, arms, shoulders, neck, and head. After relaxing all the muscle groups, spend a few moments relishing the feeling of a totally relaxed body. After some practice you may find that you do not need to tense the muscle groups first, but can relax them one by one on command.

Meditation involves clearing your mind and focusing

on one symbolic word or image or on the rhythm of your breathing.

The result is a restful, healing emptiness. Relaxation techniques require practice initially. The effort is worth it, however, because the result is a feeling of physical and mental restoration and a general sense of well-being.

FIND A SUPPORT GROUP

Joining support groups help people cope better with their conditions. There are groups that center around psychosocial issues such as grief or stress reduction. Other groups focus on the concerns of specific medical diagnoses such as arthritis, respiratory conditions, and stroke. Typically these groups have an educational component as well as a sharing of experiences. Often spouses and other family members are welcome to attend also.

Support group members learn from each other by sharing information about community resources and tips for coping. Members use their shared experiences to bolster each other during difficult periods. New members find others who truly understand the mental and physical challenges they face.

For many, support groups are the impetus to rechannel their efforts at a time when one is apt to become withdrawn. Attending group meetings means getting out of the house and meeting new people. Support groups also provide opportunities for you to help others.

Meetings are often listed in the newspaper. If you do not find them there, try asking at the library, hospital, or doctor's office. If you do not find a group for your disease or condition, consider joining another. Although your diagnosis differs from that of the other members, you may still have much to learn and to contribute.

PETS HAVE THERAPEUTIC VALUE

Stroking the fur of a gentle animal can be very restful and rewarding and the bond that develops between pet and owner seems uniquely satisfying. Animals have been shown to be very therapeutic companions.

Since pets require care it seems contradictory to recommend them in a book on energy conservation; however, we know some people with low energy who find the rewards of pet ownership outweigh the energy costs.

CALL A PRO

It is important to recognize when you need more help. Sometimes supportive friends and relaxation periods are not enough to restore your sense of emotional well-being. Low energy makes everyone feel down sometimes; but when you feel depressed all the time, you need to turn to a professional counselor. Depression is a treatable condition. In the telephone book you will find mental health centers and private therapists. If you have the symptoms of depression — difficulty sleeping, poor appetite, crying periods, and sad thoughts — call your doctor or a mental health professional. Sometimes depression is due to a chemical imbalance in the body and can be corrected with medication. Sometimes counseling is the key to feeling better.

Emotions are a natural part of life and, whether good or bad, they elicit an energy cost. Natural though they are, your emotions are under your control. You can learn to recognize the situations, people and activities that make you feel better and worse. You can train your body to relax and give you respite from stress. You can learn to ask for help with emotional issues. Chronic low energy levels affect each individual psychologically as well as physically. Your emotional response is uniquely yours so your solution must be as well. You will need to explore and experiment in order to discover your personal antidote for the blues.

My grandmother was married in 1920, during an era of great delicacy. She tells me that on the eve of her wedding, her mother gave her only one piece of advice: Take a nap every day after lunch, dear. You'll get so much more done in the afternoon.

"Nie Dam Sie"
(I Shall Not Surrender)

CONCLUSION

By planning and pacing yourself you most certainly can accomplish the things that are important to you. Wasted energy can be decreased in a variety of ways and the ever-valuable "no" used with greater ease to increase productivity in your daily life. Improved communication skills offer the chance to nourish interpersonal relationships and enhance your physical and emotional intimacy. By knowing when to ask for help, you are able to store valuable strength for safe-keeping.

A quote I read in Arthur Rubinstein's autobiography has stayed with me through the years. It is in Polish, but the translation says it all: *"Nie Dam Sie"* — I Shall Not Surrender. Do not despair the pitfalls and frustrations of mastering the art of energy conservation. Perseverance and a sense of humor will carry you through. Do not give up. Keep on *Pacing Yourself* and your quest for personal balance will be fulfilled.

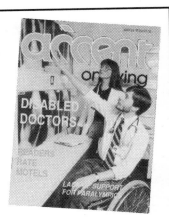
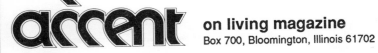